The contents of this book are for informational purposes only and do not constitute medical advice; and are not intended to be a substitute for, or replace, professional medical advice, diagnosis, or treatment. Always seek the advice of a physician or other qualified health provider with any questions you may have regarding a medical condition, and before following or relying upon any information in this book. Never disregard professional medical advice, or delay seeking it because of something you have read in this book. The author and publisher specifically disclaim any liability, loss, or risk, personal or otherwise, that is incurred as a consequence, directly or indirectly, of the use and application of any of the contents of this book.

Copyright © 2025 by Christopher Reade
This is version 001a, updated July 15th, 2025
Cover Images by Elxel Creative, Brittany Hill

The scanning, uploading, and distribution of this book without permission is a theft of the author's intellectual property. If you would like permission to use material from the book (other than for review purposes), please contact permissions@BeatingDiabetes.us. Thank you for your support of the author's rights.

LookFar Ventures
2831 Saint Claude Avenue
New Orleans LA 70117
https://BeatingDiabetes.us
Twitter.com/ BeatinDiabetes
Instagram.com/ BeatingDiabetesus
First edition: May 2025
ISBN: 979-8-9927456-0-3

The publisher is not responsible for websites (or their content) that are not owned by the publisher.

Beating Diabetes: How A Botched Insurance Renewal Saved My Life

By Christopher Reade

Contents

Part I: Background

Chapter 1: My Story - How a Botched Insurance Renewal Saved My Life

Chapter 2: Diabetes Types, Causes, and Conventional Treatments

Part II: Understanding Diabetes and Blood Sugar

Chapter 3: What A1C is and why you need to care about it

Chapter 4: Testing 1,2,3

Chapter 5: The Glycemic Index Explained

Part III: The Soluble Fiber Solution

Chapter 6: What is Soluble Fiber - Soluble Fiber's Role in Controlling Blood Sugar

Chapter 7: Sources of Soluble Fiber in Everyday Life

Chapter 8: Studies I Bet My Life On

Part IV: Practical Implementation

Chapter 9: Reading Nutrition Labels for Sugar Control

Chapter 10: Recipes that kick A$$ For Soluble Fiber

Chapter 11: How to Eat at Any Restaurant with Sugar Control in Mind

Part V: Making These Changes Stick

Chapter 12: Habit Stacking, Virtue Bundling and Concierge Doctors

Chapter 13: Stress Management and Sleep

Chapter 14: Exercise – the Great Cure-All

Part VI: Additional Considerations

Chapter 15: Alcohol and Diabetes

Chapter 16: Supplements and Alternative Treatments

Chapter 17: The Scarlet Letter D

Foreword

> "Everybody will get obsessed with their health at some point; the only question is will it be before or after your diagnosis?"

As a former Powerlifting National Champion, certified personal trainer, and nutrition coach, I've spent my life understanding the power of discipline, strategic eating, and physical health. But beyond the competition stage and the gym, I've also seen the other side—the quiet epidemic affecting millions of people, one blood sugar spike at a time. It's called pre-diabetes, and it's the point of no return for many, not because they can't turn it around, but because they don't even know they need to.

We live in a society that reacts instead of prevents, where people wait for a diagnosis before they start caring about their health. But Type 2 diabetes doesn't just arrive overnight. It's a slow, creeping condition that gives plenty of warning signs—signs that most people don't recognize until it's too late. That's why I believe so strongly in prevention and early intervention. We must work hard to help people get their health on track before it becomes a life sentence.

I have known or known of Chris for close to two decades now, and I have had a front row seat to watch his transformation. And now having read all the details in this book, I could not be any prouder of him. Here was someone who not only confronted his diagnosis head-on but found a way to turn it around—without falling into the trap of extreme dieting or a lifetime of medication. His journey is both inspiring and practical, showing that diabetes doesn't have to be progressive or incurable. It can be controlled. It can be reversed.

Chris's approach resonates deeply with me because it aligns with the philosophies I've applied throughout my career and life. Like training for a championship, it's about consistency, discipline, and smart choices. It's about making sustainable changes rather than chasing temporary fixes. Most importantly, it's about reclaiming control—taking responsibility before someone else must.

I've built and sold two wellness-based companies, coaching countless people to better health. Through that journey, I've witnessed firsthand that the most powerful transformations come not just from diet or exercise but from a mindset shift. It's about choosing health every day before you're forced to. This book provides the roadmap for that choice.

To everyone reading this, I hope this story empowers you to get obsessed with your health now, before it becomes an emergency. Let this be the wake-up call, the motivation, and the guide you need to make changes today that will save your tomorrow.

Welcome to a new way of thinking about diabetes, health, and life itself.

— Erik Frank

2010 American National Powerlifting champion
Certified Personal Trainer
Certified Nutrition Coach.
Certified Scaling Up Coach

Part 1: Background

My Friend Tim

My close friends know of my journey from when my sugar levels went suddenly off the charts in 2017 to getting my health on track a few months later. Obviously, they noticed when I dropped a quick 20 pounds and kept it off for years.

I actually started writing this book because one of them, Tim, reached out to me when his own sugar went haywire. In his case, he'd gone from "normal" or "slightly elevated" sugar levels to an A1C (the standard measure of your average blood sugar) of almost 11, with doctors wanting to either admit him to the hospital or pump him full of insulin.

He called me shortly thereafter and asked me how I did what I did. I gave him a firehose of information but soon realized there was no way I could quickly help him get up to speed without writing it down. And once I started writing my story down, I realized it made more sense to turn it into the book I'd been thinking about writing ever since I got my own sugar under control.

So, this book is thanks to Tim and is dedicated to him and to all the other people I know who are fighting to control their sugar but haven't found anyone willing to tell them straight how it really works. **It's for everyone who wants what I found: a way of life that gives them what they want – no drugs (or fewer drugs) and no progressive disease or symptoms.**

Chapter 1: My Story: How a Botched Insurance Renewal Saved My Life

This book is the story of my journey from out-of-control sugar in November of 2017 to an A1C of 5.5 less than six months later – and how a botched life insurance renewal, of all things, saved my life. It's also a practical guide showing how I keep my sugar levels under control without prescription drugs, and why I believe others can do exactly what I did without resorting to extreme diets.

First, the Botched Life Insurance Renewal

In 2017 my insurance agent moved from ABC insurance to XYZ Insurance (not their real names to keep me out of trouble). I was supposed to be assigned a new agent, but noticed something askew when I didn't receive my quarterly bill. So, I reached out to my former agent, who reminded me that he'd switched to XYZ, and my policy remained with ABC. As a favor he said he'd check with the agent who had picked up his accounts.

My former agent called me back to tell me it had been a good thing I hadn't died because ABC had really screwed up and never renewed the policy when it had come around – it was the first year of the policy. So here I was with no life insurance and a seven-year-old child and a wife who worked in our company with me. My "new" agent arranged for a new policy but now we needed to redo the medical examinations and paperwork.

At the time I didn't think anything of it. I've always been a healthy person, and I play a lot of volleyball, and I ski and surf, so I figured, *why worry?* The worst that had ever shown up in my medical history was being a little overweight (196 the day of the test) and slightly elevated cholesterol. I had heard the term A1C but I didn't know what it meant. When the blood work came back, and my blood sugar was at 150 or 175 and my A1C was at 9.1, I figured it was just a bad test – I had ignored the fasting instructions and had a piece of cake the evening before. I told my agent this was crazy, and we should re-do the test. He suggested I go see a doctor first and see what was up.

Potential Diagnosis

I didn't even have a regular physician at that time – my doctor had retired a few years earlier and I'd never bothered to find a new one. As I mentioned, the blood tests from just a year earlier had shown me to be in really good shape.

When I found a new doctor the next week, she took a look at the tests and said, "Here's a prescription for Metformin, and if that doesn't work well enough, we'll get you on insulin."

""Insulin?!? What the hell…" I said. "I don't want to be on meds the rest of my life."

She said flatly, "Diabetes is an incurable, progressive disease – you will have it the rest of your life."

"I don't have diabetes," I said.

Her response: "Let's test it again in a couple months – but for now let's treat it like it's diabetes."

I left her office determined to find another way. But I did get that prescription filled.

I read as many studies as I could on the various ways people have tried to control diabetes. I researched how to get your pancreas to manufacture more insulin again. And I discovered crucial pieces of information that ultimately led me to a sustainable way of life that controls sugar and has eliminated diabetes for me.

This book is about that way of life.

In many ways that original doctor was right – even though I don't show up diabetic on any tests and never have had an A1C over 5.7 since that first one, I still watch my sugar intake at every meal and use an at-home A1C test quarterly to make sure things are still good. And here I am writing a book about it.

But while that doctor was right, she was leaving out something crucial that many physicians aren't aware of – you can actually eliminate diabetes, or at least certainly push it into remission (your choice of terms). This has been studied extensively since the '70s and really isn't controversial, even though it is mostly ignored by the medical establishment. Most of what's in this book comes from those studies and their modern counterparts that I read and then put into practice.

Examining the Options and the Evidence

So, what did I do? Well, as I mentioned above, I read and researched the heck out of the options. I also got some professional help on my side – experts who helped me figure out how to live without prescription drugs while still controlling my blood sugar and A1C. Two important first stops on my journey were a nutritionist and finding a doctor willing to work with me.

Concierge Doctors

Concierge doctors are a godsend, it turns out. If you can afford one, it is definitely worth the investment. A "regular" doctor will almost certainly be uninterested in helping you figure out how to control a "progressive" and "incurable" disease without drugs because they just have too many patients and not enough time. With a concierge doctor, you're literally paying them to work with you and find solutions.

I'll get into the details later about how to find a concierge doctor, how to tell if they're right for you, and what the costs typically run. But the point I want to make here is this: <u>Having a medical</u>

<u>professional in your corner who actually wants to help you solve the problem – rather than just writing prescriptions – is incredibly valuable.</u>

Nutritionists

I also tried working with a nutritionist, but frankly, I found it wasn't worth the time and energy. I actually ended up being more educated about soluble fiber and its effects on metabolism than several of the nutritionists I spoke to about these topics. <u>This isn't to say they won't be helpful for people trying to replicate what I did to beat diabetes – they might be great for you. But for me, the time spent working with them just wasn't worth it.</u>

My Process – My Way of Living

In the simplest terms, my process can be broken down into three areas of activity that combine to control sugar levels. My process also led to losing 10% of my body weight. The American Diabetes Association recommends that a weight loss of 7% to 10% can help prevent disease progression, which is a nice thing to say but I really wish they would come out and say what they know, which is that losing 10% of your body weight often pushes diabetes into remission all by itself.[1]

For me, I did the following things, and this has eliminated diabetes completely from my life. I still do these things, and they have allowed me to get rid of prescription medications from my daily routine.

> 1 – **I became very educated on what metabolizes as sugar and why.** I also regularly look up the glucose index (GI) of foods if I am not sure.

---

[1] See ADA guidelines ("Lose weight for good") and other articles at https://diabetes.org/health-wellness/weight-management

2 – **I learned about the power of soluble or dietary fiber** - I use this type of fiber to balance out what I eat that does metabolize into sugar.

3 – **I do not deprive myself of all sweets or all carbs, etc.** I have birthday cake but when I do I make sure to load up on soluble fiber shortly or immediately beforehand and I eat a smaller slice than I used to. I never "diet" – study after study shows that dieting ends almost everyone up right back where they were before they started.

I'll explain more about each of these in turn later in this book.

Dieting – or, more precisely, not dieting.

I don't think "diets" are a good thing. I'll share some studies later in this book that show why I think dieting is a terrible idea – something that exists mainly to sell us stuff and keep us jumping from one fad to another. But here's what's important: I'm not pushing a "diet" here. Instead, I'm offering a way to think about what you eat so you never have to "diet" again. The methods I'm championing aren't some temporary fix – they're a way of life that, once you get into it, becomes almost effortless.

Studies

In Part III I cite and review what I learned from various studies so that you can read them for yourself and see why I took away from them what I did. In the United States there has not historically been a lot of research on reversing diabetes because there is huge economic gain and interest in keeping people diabetic.

Diabetes is just too profitable for too many parties and its status as "progressive," and "incurable" is unchallenged by our medical establishment here. The UK, Canada and some other European countries have the best studies on the subject. This is probably because they have single-payer health systems where the incentive is strong to get people off meds and to reverse diabetes.

Chapter 2: Diabetes Types, Causes, and Conventional Treatments

Diabetes is a disease that occurs when your blood glucose, aka sugar, is chronically too high. Glucose is necessary for most things that your body does – it is your body's main source of energy. Your body both makes glucose and also takes it directly from the food you eat.

Insulin is a hormone made by your pancreas that helps glucose get into your cells so you can use it for energy. However, if there is too much sugar in your blood, your body needs to make insulin, which binds to the sugar and locks it away from harming your organs. Diabetes means that your body doesn't make <u>enough</u> (type 2) — or <u>any</u> (type 1) —insulin or doesn't use insulin properly. Glucose then stays in your blood and doesn't reach your cells. This results in organ damage over time.

Diabetes raises the risk for damage to the eyes, kidneys, nerves, and heart. Diabetes is also linked to some types of cancer.[2] According to the United States National Institutes of Health, *"Diabetes (primarily type 2) is associated with increased risk for some cancers (liver, pancreas, endometrium, colon and rectum, breast, bladder)."*

---

[2] Please see "Diabetes and Cancer: A consensus report" at
https://pmc.ncbi.nlm.nih.gov/articles/PMC2890380/

Type 1 vs Type 2

Type 1 diabetes is of unknown provenance generally but has genetic components and environmental ones - but whatever causes it, the effect is that your immune system attacks and kills your islet cells, which are the parts of your pancreas that create and secrete insulin into your bloodstream. This renders your body unable to make insulin at all. A small percentage of people with diabetes are type 1 – between 5 and 10% depending on which stats you check. Most people are type 2.

For type 2 diabetics the immune system is not involved, and it appears to be fat in or on your pancreas that causes the islet cells to underperform.[3] Specifically, "This type of fat, called visceral fat, causes inflammation and insulin resistance and is strongly linked with cardiovascular disease.[4]

As noted above, islet cells are the cells in your pancreas that manufacture insulin for you. But in almost all type 2 diabetics, the islet cells do work somewhat, just not enough to control blood sugar on their own. This is why type 2 is "progressive." If unchecked, this process means that more and more of your islet cells stop working or work partially and you need bigger interventions, like going from just taking metformin pills to having to take insulin shots.

It is thought, and there is evidence for the idea, that losing 10% of body weight works because you wring out the fat from the pancreas, but while this has been shown to be true in some studies it is not a 100% accepted orthodoxy. As noted above, visceral fat causes inflammation and insulin resistance and is strongly linked with cardiovascular disease.

How to lose fat in a particular spot is impossible currently, but would obviously be amazing for many reasons. It is thought that the issue of small

---

[3] See Chapter 8 and the Direct Study at
https://www.ncl.ac.uk/magres/research/diabetes/reversal/#publicinformation
[4] See "What causes the insulin resistance underlying obesity?"
https://pmc.ncbi.nlm.nih.gov/articles/PMC4038351/

amounts of "visceral" fat on the pancreas is why some obese people never become diabetic and why some very active, otherwise healthy people do – the skinny folks are unlucky and gain fat in an unfortunate spot - their pancreas. While people with a much higher body fat percentage might not ever store fat on their pancreas and thus never become type 2 diabetics, despite being obese.

It is important to note that while the way of living I am describing in this book would help a person who has type 1 diabetes, it wouldn't keep them from needing insulin via shots or pills. Type 1 is an immune issue ultimately, and while soluble fiber can help control sugar spikes for people with type 1, it isn't up to the job of doing so as a complete solution for that kind of diabetes.

Personally, I've never hit that magical number of fat cells that would get my pancreas to function at 100% again. However, it definitely does function, and I have definitely increased that function with good soluble-fiber-centric eating. But for a person with Type 1 diabetes, the immune system kills off the islet cells if they start functioning again, even in transplant patients.[5] This is a fascinating problem and studied extensively because many chronic diseases like MS or Type 1 diabetes are a huge and currently unsolvable issue.

Concierge Doctors

I am acutely aware of the privilege I had in my journey to "Beating Diabetes" - that I was able to afford testing kits, experimental foods, nutritionists and a concierge doctor. I could just say that "I worked my butt off all of my adult life and thank God I did so and that it paid off enough to save my life later." But I also was lucky, lucky, lucky in so many ways. Lastly, the truth is that most of the things I have outlined here in this book aren't as expensive as they sound. One of those things is a concierge doctor.

---

[5] See the 2023 study by the NIH at https://pmc.ncbi.nlm.nih.gov/articles/PMC10000424/

But what is a "Concierge Doctor"?

In the simplest sense of the phrase, a concierge doctor is a primary care physician whom you pay some set amount to on some schedule (monthly, quarterly, etc.) directly for easier access. This is a pretty symbiotic relationship in that the doctor gets to have fewer patients and much less overhead because they aren't dealing with insurance companies. They also get more time with patients and the satisfaction of feeling like they really help people – and they do!

For the patient, you get access to a doctor you can just call or email and make an appointment whenever you want or, within reason, as many times a year as you need to. When I first signed up with my concierge doctor, I went and saw her monthly. I was able to sit down and explain to her what I was trying to do, and she was able to help guide me towards things that might work and things to avoid.

As the years have gone on, I see her much less - but when I need her, she's there immediately. Which is what you really want out of the medical establishment at the end of the day – someone who actually listens to your issues and is available when you need them.

The other key thing about concierge docs is that they also can prescribe, just like any other doctor, but without the red tape and often can get the meds themselves in their office so you don't even go to the CVS or Walgreens and might even save a couple bucks.

Lastly, just like other primary care physicians, concierge doctors are gatekeepers to specialists and usually know many of them. For example, about a year ago I had a bad reaction to some very expired sunscreen and gave myself chemical burns all over my face and neck. She was able to give me some basic meds but, more importantly, she was able to get me in with a dermatologist the next day. They can't always do that kind of stuff for you, but if it's important, you can bet they'll try their best.

Ok, great, so how much $ are we talking here?

I don't want to give away trade secrets here, but I did my research before I picked this particular doctor, and they all seemed to land around the price of a cable bill or a mobile phone bill. Your mileage may vary as they say. Mine, for example, charges quarterly and I can use my HSA to pay for it. Others may only do a credit card and charge monthly.

My advice here is to ask around, do your internet research and meet with several potential doctors or at least talk to their RN (most seem to have one whom is in charge of their office). They typically have smaller offices since they see fewer people. Many have a TeleMed option where you can talk with them over Zoom or something similar.

Part II: Understanding Diabetes and Blood Sugar

Chapter 3: What A1C is and why you need to care about it

As the great Yogi Berra once said, *"You've got to be very careful if you don't know where you are going, because you might not get there."* It's not possible to know when you've gotten your blood sugar under control if you don't define what "under control" means and what "reversing diabetes" means.

A1C essentially means the average amount of glucose floating around in your blood. The extra sugar that isn't being trapped for processing by insulin is what damages your organs and causes health troubles. Since A1C represents an average, it takes about 30 days to "change" much. Personally, I check it at home every three to four months (see Chapter 4 where I discuss home tests and other paraphernalia).

Below and to the right are several A1C charts. The first is from the Cleveland Clinic, the second from GoodRx, and the third

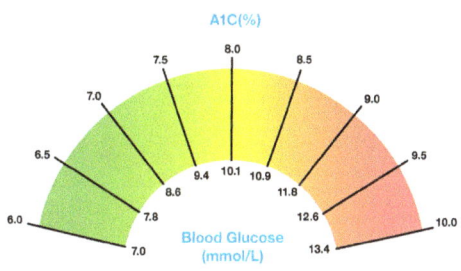

BEATING DIABETES

from Diabetes Care Community. Notice that the "Normal" level is a relative statement.

Mostly you will see 5.7 as the "magic" number to get under, but many places will tell you that anything less than 6.3 is "no action" or nothing to worry about. I would consider anything under 5.7 an indication of diabetes in remission and anything over that an indication that more work needs to be done. That doesn't mean a person following the path I took would get there immediately – it took me about 4-6 months to really get things under control.

Spikiness

What A1C is really telling you is how often your sugar spikes – meaning how often it goes over 150+.[6] This is the active part of diabetes and why it is a dangerous disease. Those spikes/highs make you feel like crap in the short term – lethargic, slow and dull because of what is called "oxidative stress."[7] In the long term, repeated spikes in your blood sugar **can cause heart problems, kidney problems, problems with eyesight, gum disease, and nerve issues like neuropathy**, where you lose feeling in fingers and toes.

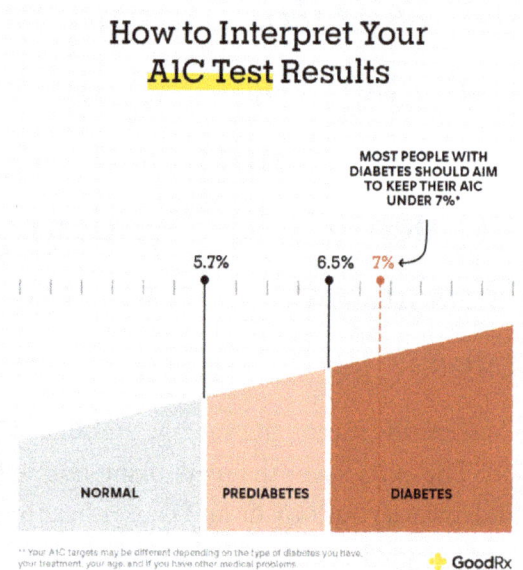

---

[6] See "High Morning Blood Glucose: Understanding and Management" https://diabetes.org/living-with-diabetes/high-morning-blood-glucose
[7] See "Why are blood sugar spikes bad for us?" at https://www.tryhabitual.com/journal/why-are-blood-sugar-spikes-bad-for-us

In my experience, I was able to drop my A1C from 9-ish to 6 in 45 days and have never had it over 5.7 in over 7 years and counting. So, if I was to advise someone on what goal they should have for their A1C level, I'd say "don't get excited until you get under 6 – and the goal is under 5.7."

There's a lot of different information about what "normal" means. For example, in the chart shown from **GoodRx**, you see that "Most people with diabetes should aim to keep their A1C under 7%." I understand what they're trying to say here, but for me, if you are a diabetic and you're on insulin or one of the insulin-like drugs, you should be aiming for an A1C of under 5.7, because that is, after all, what you are taking powerful drugs for in the first place.

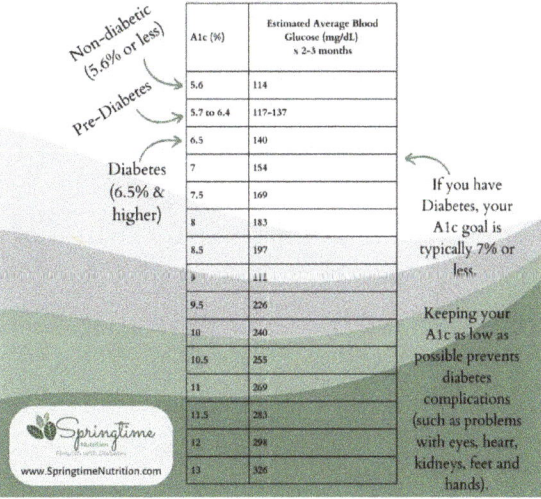

But the way this reads it makes it seem like 7% is "normal" for diabetics. Maybe that would be "normal" for diabetics without control over their sugar levels, but I think we do people a disservice when we give them targets to hit that aren't actually good for them. For what I've read, 7% is too high to avoid long-term health issues and it's definitely too high if you're taking insulin.

Here again we have a chart with the same information (this one from Springtime Nutrition[8]), but in a slightly different format. This one does the conversion from "A1C to Blood Sugar," which usually can be taken to mean fasting or morning blood sugar readings (more on that later).

---

[8] See original chart at https://springtimenutrition.com/a1c-conversion-chart/

All of these charts and the thousands of others you can find online tell you not to take any action under 6.5 and start food restriction and medication if it gets over 8.

It is my position that if your A1C is 9 it's more than high time to start "food restriction" – and if your A1C is over 12 most doctors that I have spoken with would send you to a hospital.

The point here is that you will see these charts in a thousand different formats and presentations, but they all say roughly the same things. And that is pretty much what the NIH and other authorities say – **keep your A1C at 5.7 or less** and you'll probably never have a problem with sugar-related health issues. That certainly is low enough to avoid most if not all complications of high blood sugar and diabetes.

Chapter 4 - Testing 1,2,3…

There's only one thing more important than knocking your A1C and glucose levels down to normal or nearly normal, and that is <u>knowing</u> that you did and that you continue to knock down these levels. And the only way you can really know this is to test. But as with everything in life, there are potential complications you need to consider when thinking about tests.

At first, I tested my fasting blood sugar every day for glucose levels. After a few years of seeing them largely stay the same, anywhere from 98 on the low-side to 115 on the high-side when I wake up, I lowered the frequency.

I got to a place where my morning blood sugar just wasn't changing that much after about a year, and I slowly backed off of daily and went to bi-weekly and then monthly. The thing I was looking for was equilibrium and general balance.

Anyone who has seen a Continuous Monitor's output (like a Dexcom™) knows that blood sugar is literally changing from minute to minute, which is one of the many reasons that **A1C is the better guidepost for your progress**. Broadly speaking, your blood sugar is highest when you first wake up in the morning, which is why insurance tests mandate that your testing be done with "fasting."

This is because, as weird as this sounds, your liver produces sugar from the food you eat – in fact, it produces a great deal of the sugar circulating around in your blood and sometimes causes spikes itself.[9] That is what metformin and berberine do – they tell the liver to chill out and make less sugar.

It's also why alcohol is dangerous to type 1 and out-of-control type 2 diabetics – not because it metabolizes as sugar but because it occupies your liver's functions and can make your blood sugar drop dangerously. In other words, alcohol <u>does not</u> metabolize as sugar, full stop. What it does do is depress your liver's function of creating glucose and thus is dangerous if your sugar is out of control like in type 1 diabetes or severe type 2.

Testing every day is a must when you are trying to get things under control. It's great to see those numbers fall from 150-ish like when I started, down to the 90s and low 100s. This positive feedback helps you realize that you are accomplishing something. It also gives you a sense of what's going on with your body in a "point in time" way, which I think is really important for giving yourself motivation to continue to improve. Meaning that it gives you these single data points at given intervals (every morning for most people) and these act as a guide for whether things are going well or poorly. I think it is too much data and "analysis paralysis" to use minute-by-minute devices like Dexcom's – they also cost a lot of $ relative to test strips.

---

[9] See "How The Liver Influences Your Sugar Metabolism"
https://www.mysugr.com/en/blog/how-liver-influences-your-sugar-metabolism

Test Strips and Devices

The basics of point-in-time glucose testing are a small device that can "see" how much sugar is in a blood sample and a "test strip," which is a small strip of paper with an embedded diode on which you put a drop of blood. You use a small lancet device to make a very small prick, typically at the end of a finger, which is just large enough to get a drop of blood from.

In the simplest description, you take the test strip and put it in the device. Then you use the lancet device to prick your finger. Place your finger on the end of the test strip and voila! the sample gets sucked onto the active part of the test strip. The measuring device "thinks" for a count of five or so and then displays the glucose level in the sample.

As you might imagine, there are a whole lot of brands and styles of these devices, lancets, etc. I'll go into my favorites below, but the point here is that they all work pretty much the same and they all tell you one thing – what is the current glucose level in my blood?

Now, I know an elderly man who is an uncontrolled diabetic, complete with twice daily insulin shots and lots of medical issues around high and low sugar, including some hospital visits. Somehow, he can walk and talk at 400 glucose. That would, at a minimum, put you or me into a hospital. But somehow it doesn't affect him the same way. I have another friend who works hard to control her sugar levels with meds but doesn't utilize soluble fiber. For her, a reading over 200 and she's ready to pass out.

Because we are humans and not machines, every individual has different set points for bad outcomes from sugar levels, but the key thing to remember is that you want to keep your sugar level at or below 100 ideally. I can't seem to do that regularly myself, even though my A1C is normal to low.

Your mileage may vary considerably here, as the kids say. While daily glucose monitoring is a great tool and can help you figure your levels, it's your A1C level that really tells the story you care about. This is especially true when you're first trying to get things under control.

It is "spikes" in your blood sugar level that damages your organs and makes your teeth fall out and gives you neuropathy, etc., and that's what A1C is measuring and why insurance companies and endocrinologists care so much about it. We'll get into that kind of testing next.

Glucose Testing Kits

As noted above, glucose kits have four components – a testing device (typically with an embedded battery that will last for years), testing strips that you put blood on, a lancet or finger-pricker, and disposable lancets.

It is important to note that the test strips and the measuring device must go together but you can use whatever lancet (and matching disposable lancet cartridges) you want – blood is blood, after all. I also found that the little carrying case from one system I tried was best, so I keep the lancets and the device in a nice little pouch that holds them all conveniently even though none of the items in it are the ones it came with. The point is: make it easy for yourself to test glucose because at the end of the day, ease of use equals use.

Lancets

The lancet device in a test kit is typically the most annoying part. This is because you must insert a new cartridge into it to prick your finger safely – for obvious sanitation reasons you wouldn't want to reuse such a device. A reused one would also contaminate your readings potentially, which would defeat the point of doing them.

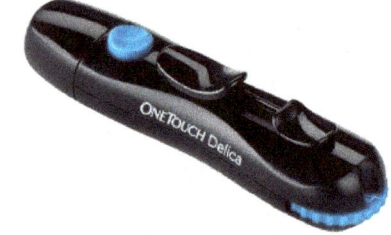

Brands
OneTouch Delica

OneTouch Delica is my go-to on the glucose test system. The lancets are the easiest for me to deal with and there are cheap generic lancets that work just fine in it.

It looks like OneTouch is replacing this unit with a "plus" version. I'm sure it costs more but hopefully it works as well.

Microlet Next

I've used this one when I was first fighting my sugar level and testing constantly.

It works fine and gets the job done but it's a bit bulky as you can see from the picture, and I wouldn't ever use it in place of the Delica one.

AUVON Lancing Device

This is one I've seen at my father's assisted living facility. The thing I like about it is what you see in the image to your right where it shoots out the used lancet. Even with my favorite, the Delica OneTouch, it is annoying to get the lancet out of the device and into the trash.

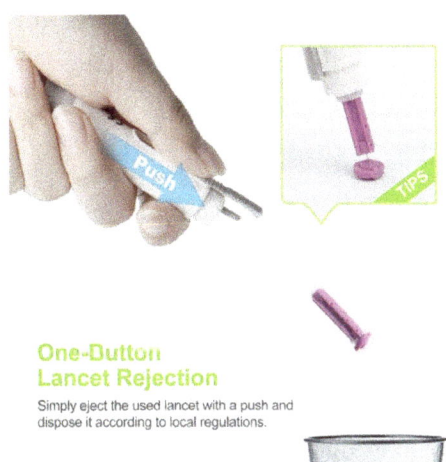

One-Button Lancet Rejection

Simply eject the used lancet with a push and dispose it according to local regulations.

I imagine the RNs at my dad's facility started using it because it lets you avoid accidental needle sticks, which are annoying but not hazardous when it's your own blood but is an issue when you're in a healthcare facility.

<u>At the end of the day, all the lancet devices are annoying to use. In my experience, the OneTouch Delica is the least annoying.</u>

Testers, aka Glucose Meters

So, the lancets are how you get blood out of your body in order to test it, typically by pricking your finger. The tester is an electronic device that can "see" sugar on specially designed little test strips. This has a shaving blade type market – typically the testing devices are cheaper than you'd expect them to be, but they get you on the test strips, which you can generally only buy from the manufacturer. There are some generic strips but it's hard to know if they're as accurate as the ones from the company that makes the device, so I tend to stick with the brand-name here.

Brands

Contour Next One Blood Glucose Meter

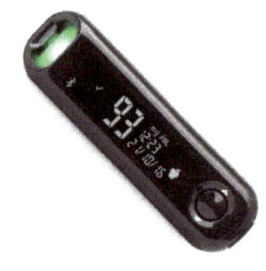

This is the one I've been using for years. It's fast, accurate and the strips won't set you back a fortune. What's not to love? The one thing I note when I go look for images of this tester is that it is hilarious and aspirational at best to have a 93 displayed on the screen – the people buying this are not likely throwing down 93 blood sugar levels!

OneTouch® Ultra® 2 meter

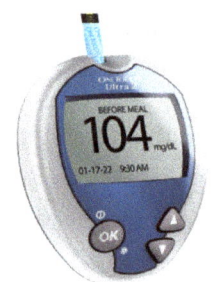

This is one I used when I first got the Delica lancet device, and I was trying to stay in the same "family" of products. It's fine as meters go – I just didn't love the size of this device which is a pretty minor dislike, but when you use something every day you want it to be small and convenient.

Generic testers and "Wi-Fi" connected ones

Professionally I am a technologist. I run a software company, I was a computer programmer by training, and I was certified in various network technologies. So, I am professionally paranoid about data, and I don't like devices with sensitive medical information hooked up to Wi-Fi. I realize that this puts me on the outside edge of comfort level, but I avoid Wi-Fi connected medical devices if at all possible.

Generic Walmart, CVS, Walgreens, etc. brand glucose testers are all fine in my book. They might work just as well as the ones I've had for years that I outlined above, but there is definitely a "you get what you pay for" thing going on here as well.

A1C Home Tests

Before the medical people start screaming at me and throwing this book across the room, I'll own up to knowing perfectly well that a home A1C test is not as good as one done in a lab. That said, the home kits I've used are pretty darn good and they really help me out a lot because I can do the test without making an appointment at a Quest Diagnostics place or similar.

Typically speaking, most insurance companies will pay for one set of blood work a year. That's simply not good enough for me and it shouldn't be for you. I want to know that I'm on track and so paying out of pocket for a lab test because just doing it once a year will not get the job done.

Nowadays I use the home test kits about every 4 months or so, but when I first started this journey, I used them monthly and paid for the lab tests quarterly because I was trying my darndest to prove that I could control sugar and beat diabetes – I don't suggest you do it that way as it's a lot of work and probably gives you more data than is useful – things just don't change that fast.

The home test kit I use, which you can get from many places online, is **PTS Diagnostics' A1C Now Test Kit** with 4 tests per box.[10] Now, there are some picadilloes to this test kit that I will go into below but overall, it works great and after I learned how to use it, I almost never waste a test, and it matches nearly 100% to my lab tests. If anything, it's a bit higher reading

---

[10] See https://www.totaldiabetessupply.com/products/a1c-now-4-test-kit and https://www.ptsdiagnostics.com/a1cnow-self-check/

than the lab tests. If a test is going to have any disagreement with a lab test, I'd want it to be in that direction anyway.

The directions to these kits, like pretty much everything like this in the world, are uniformly terrible. This kit at least has reasonably decent diagrams to help you.

The part about using this kit that I have found annoying and has caused me to waste kits (the "regular" size comes with six test kits), is the blood sample device. Now, I can totally understand that this is the hardest part of the whole process – it's the part where we're dealing with a human bodily fluid and trying to get an average person to accurately get the sample on their own with zero training and just one badly-written instruction guide to help them. But does it have to be this hard to get the right amount of blood?!

Most of the time when I screwed this up originally, I didn't get enough blood in it (works out to roughly two drops). But because it is a totally clear tube with a clear reservoir at the bottom, it's really hard to see how much is enough. And if you go the other way and keep adding more, your test will fail because of over-sampling.

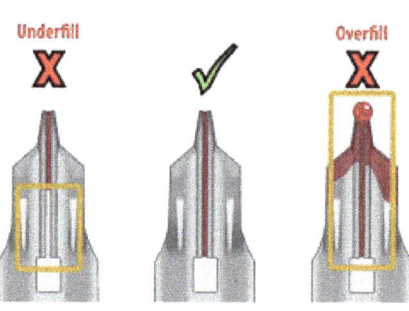

The picture here is what it looks like when you get this "right." If any blood is over the top of the little suction tube, you will get an error. If the tube isn't filled to the top, you will get an error. Once you do it a few times you'll get the hang of it. But take heart – you are hardly the only one on the struggle bus with this device. Just Google it up and you'll see.

But once you get the blood sample out of the way the rest of the process is super simple, and you get a pretty accurate A1C reading in 5 minutes. Total cost per test (I figure I screw one up per box) works out to about $15-20 or about $65 for four.

And, because I am a paranoic techie, I also like that this test is not hooked up to any systems and is not available to anyone who isn't in the room when I do the test. This comes into play in the Chapter I call **How Personal is Personal? The Scarlet Letter "D."**

Dexcom or Continuous Glucose Monitoring

Dexcom makes a small device that attaches to your upper arm and stays on there for about ten days. It is then replaced with a new one. This device pairs with your phone and/or to a dedicated reader to tell you what your blood sugar level is (and was) pretty much all of the time. You can get cool graphs (example below), and it alerts you if your sugar gets below or above certain levels that you can set but come preset to reasonable levels.

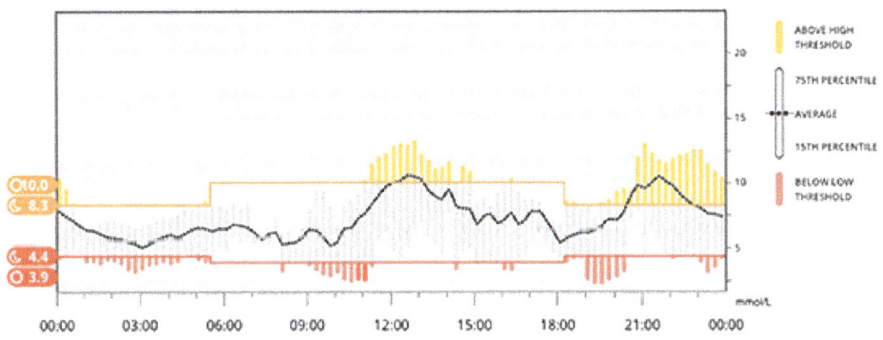

For type 1 diabetics this is a godsend, because the other option is to prick their fingers before and/or after every meal. As a friend of mine said when his nine-year old came down with type 1, the school nurse and he are now close friends. Type 1 is much harder to manage, and you can't really control it or push it into remission at the time of this writing.

Dexcoms and similar can be useful for someone trying to control their sugar using the methods outlined in this book, but I worry that it will become a crutch and I'm against them generally. It's also annoying to change the arm device every ten days, I don't like things on my body, and I also got on this path to get rid of medical interventions, not invite them into my life on a perpetual basis. Also, as a technologist, I know perfectly well that using a Dexcom or similar is feeding data to my insurance carrier on a minute-by-minute basis, and I don't like that creepy stuff at all.

One solid use case I have seen in friends who have them is to utilize a Dexcom for a few months to see what really moves your sugar. Every human body is slightly different and responds to things a little differently. For some people potatoes may only jack their sugar a little bit but rice will spike them big time. **I would still argue that the Glycemic Index is a better long-term tool, especially because it is free, but using a Dexcom or similar for this purpose seems reasonable to me.**

All this is to say, if someone who was trying to control their sugar told me they were using a Dexcom I'd say, "if it helps you out then use it." I'm a big believer in what the 12-step programs say on this subject – "take what you need, leave the rest."

Summary

Testing is important – especially when you're first getting your sugar under control and beating back diabetes into remission. Daily glucose tests are a great tool to help you build a habit of thinking about your sugar and what your goals are.

But in the end, it is the change in the way I approach food and live that does the trick in the long run. It's not daily testing, which I rarely do anymore, that keeps my A1C and sugar levels balanced – it's how I eat, exercise and live. It's the habit-stacking and virtue-bundling that's doing the real work. The tests just tell me the process is working, which is critical, but it is not the end goal. Beating diabetes and making sure it never comes back into my life is the end goal.

Chapter 5: The Glycemic Index Explained

The greatest human accomplishments in medicine, technology and pretty much every applied science field come from the Scientific Method. As you may recall from high school, a big part of the scientific process is having controls and strongly researched references. This is where the Glycemic Index comes from and why it matters and is useful.

The scientists who study food for its nutritional value, effects on the body and other purposes created the glycemic index to allow for foods to be compared to each other based on what happens in your metabolism when you consume them – how much glucose/sugar they create. For "normal" people who just want to figure out if they should eat something, this is a godsend. I refer to it at least weekly nowadays and I used to check it daily for what I was eating.

Glycemic Index

Because diabetes is so prevalent, there is an agreed upon way to measure the amount of sugar in various foods. This is published online in a ton of places so that you can literally google up "GI Index [insert food]" and you'll get an intelligible number back. Originally created by a scientist named Dr. David Jenkins at the University of Toronto in 1980-1981, this way of categorizing food has been a staple of sugar control ever since.[11]

> The short version of the chart below is that foods under 50 GI are "good". I argue that 40 is a better "good" point for people trying to control sugar levels.

I use Google as a guide if I'm not sure of the glycemic index of a particular food. My personal favorite, as with many things in this book, is the British NHS list and one from the UK's Diabetes Organization[12] that works to get their government to take it more seriously. Frankly though, Google is the easiest way to do this quickly, like looking at nutrition labels at the grocery store. There's an example of one of these lists below (this one is from Very Well Health), but you can literally find hundreds of versions online easily.

---

[11] See David Jenkins Bio at https://nutrisci.med.utoronto.ca/faculty/david-jenkins
[12] See https://www.diabetes.org.uk/guide-to-diabetes/enjoy-food/carbohydrates-and-diabetes/glycaemic-index-and-diabetes

Low-GI Foods (55 or Less)		Medium-GI Foods (56 to 69)		High-GI Foods (70 to 100)	
Foods	*GI*	*Foods*	*GI*	*Foods*	*GI*
Apple	36	Brown rice, boiled	68	Cornflakes	81
Apple juice	41	Couscous	65	Instant oatmeal	79
Banana	51	French fries	63	Potato, boiled	78
Barley	28	Millet porridge	67	Potatoes, instant mashed	87
Carrots, boiled	39	Muesli	57	Rice milk	86
Chapatti	52	Pineapple	59	Rice porridge	78
Chickpeas	28	Popcorn	65	Rice crackers	87
Chocolate	40	Potato chips	56	Unleavened wheat bread	70
Dates	42	Pumpkin, boiled	64	Watermelon	76
Ice cream	51	Soda, non-diet	59	White rice, boiled	73
Kidney beans	24	Sweet potato, boiled	63	White bread (wheat)	75
Lentils	32	Wheat flake biscuits cereal	69	Whole wheat bread	74
Mango	51	Wheat roti	62		
Orange	43				
Orange juice	50				
Plantain	55				
Rolled oats	55				
Low-GI Foods (55 or Less)		**Medium-GI Foods (56 to 69)**		**High-GI Foods (70 to 100)**	
Skim milk	37				
Soya beans	16				
Soy milk	34				
Spaghetti, white	49				
Spaghetti, whole grain	48				
Sweet corn	52				

BEATING DIABETES

Taro, boiled	53			
Udon noodles	55			
Vegetable soup	48			
Whole milk	39			
Yogurt, fruit	41			

Note: this glycemic index chart is an amalgam of several online ones that I stitched together to cover a wider variety of foods

Checking the glycemic index of foods really helps when you're first starting out on the journey to control sugar and Beat Diabetes. Thanks to checking so frequently on Google or online lists, I "know" most foods and where they land on the GI (often called the GI Index despite the redundancy in terms).

Limitations or Exceptions of the Glycemic Index

While the glycemic index is a great thing, it does have foods listed on it with low-GI values that I wouldn't touch without a strong dietary fiber source to help out with the sugar processing. An interesting example of this is pasta.

As you can read in Chapter 8, a study in the late 1970s revealed that soluble fiber slows digestion and controls sugar spikes. While this study and its implications were promptly ignored by the medical establishment, it is the key to understanding the glycemic index as you can see below.

In the study, titled "Dietary fibres, fibre analogues, and glucose tolerance: importance of viscosity," guar-gum, which is super high in soluble fiber, was taken from its natural state (where it showed a remarkable ability to control blood sugar) to a less soluble form. In the process this largely eliminated the effect on blood sugar.[13] Meaning they took the ultimate soluble fiber product, guar gum, and turned it into something that was worthless for sugar control. This shows that it is the solubility or "gumminess" of the foods that we eat that controls sugar uptake.

And this is essentially what happens with pasta. When you cook pasta, you change the structure of the starches to make them digestible (hard uncooked

---

[13] As noted in the Chapter on Studies, please see
https://pmc.ncbi.nlm.nih.gov/articles/PMC1604761/

pasta ain't great to eat, after all). If you keep it a little al dente and don't cook it to death, pasta has a low glycemic index. But if you turn it into mush, it has a very high GI just as you would expect from something that is pretty much entirely white processed flour.

"Cooking is chemistry" is an old saw but it is totally accurate and important in terms of controlling sugar. Carrots and many other veggies are best when cooked a bit but not to death, just like pasta. We're looking for a texture that is solid and palatable but not hard and not mush – that's the general marker of soluble fiber in foods.

As we'll review in the next section, the amount of soluble fiber is directly correlated to its glycemic index number.

An important note about the glycemic index. There is some variability in this. It's usually just a few points, but you do see differences depending on source and who's doing the testing. For example, I cite chickpeas below – I've seen them listed everywhere from 26 to 30.

Glycemic Load

There is a related concept called glycemic load.[14] I quote the Wikipedia article here: "The glycemic load (GL) of food is a number that estimates how much the food will raise a person's blood glucose level after it is eaten." Basically, you can take the GL number and that means the effect of one gram of pure glucose.

The idea is to take into account the speed with which different foods turn into sugar as they metabolize. I find GL a confusing number because it's hard to work out serving sizes versus grams of glucose. For example, an apple has a GL of 10. But which apple? They vary in size dramatically and have different effects.

---

[14] See https://en.wikipedia.org/wiki/Glycemic_load and https://en.wikipedia.org/wiki/Glycemic_index

I like glycemic index a lot better because it just gives me a reference value I can use to understand if a food is a "good idea" or a "bad idea."

List of Low and High GI Foods

Here is a smattering of high and low glycemic index foods and why they are listed the way they are.

Chickpeas   GI 28

Hummus, falafel and its friends are not only superstars of the soluble fiber world but unsurprisingly are very low on the glycemic index.
Photo credit: Wikimedia Commons[15]

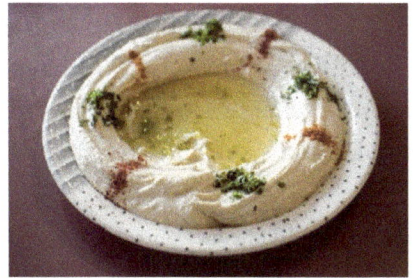

Black Beans   GI 30

Who doesn't love refried black beans? Or black bean soup? Delicious and found on practically every Mexican or Central American restaurant menu, black beans rock.

Grapefruit   GI 25

The yummy breakfast food beloved by millions. Cut in half and sliced up along the edges. It's delicious, good for you and has a super-low GI, showing that fruits certainly make the list.

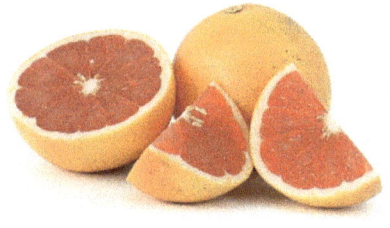

Photo credit: Wikimedia Commons[16]

---

[15] Wikimedia Commons "Hummus from The Nile.jpg"
https://commons.wikimedia.org/wiki/File:Hummus_from_The_Nile.jpg
[16] Wikimedia Commons "Citrus paradisi (Grapefruit, pink)"
https://commons.wikimedia.org/wiki/File:Citrus_paradisi_(Grapefruit,_pink)_white_bg.jpg

Bananas   GI 47

The delicious ripe banana has a relatively high GI, probably because its softness means it digests quickly. I love bananas but I rarely eat them anymore because their GI is higher than most things I eat. Some nutritionists say they're fine and I can't say I totally avoid them but there are just better fruit options for sugar control.

Bagel, White GI 65

I love, love, love bagels (I grew up in New York). But all that white bread is no good for me anymore, so I have to pass on these even though it hurts. The cream cheese is probably not terrible for sugar control and the butter is neutral, but it's still a no-go nowadays.

Photo credit: Wikimedia Commons[17]

Mashed Potatoes GI 83

At Thanksgiving I just go for it and eat a bunch of this stuff. I just love it too much to completely say no. But the rest of the year I give it a pass because the 83 GI means it's pretty much certain to spike my blood sugar.

Rice, Rice and 'Mo Rice

Photo credit: Wikimedia Commons[18]

---

[17] See Wikimedia Commons "Plain Bagel"
https://commons.wikimedia.org/wiki/File:Plain_bagel_(2884521776).jpg
[18] See Wikimedia Commons "Rice in a Bowl"
https://commons.wikimedia.org/wiki/File:Rice_In_A_Bowl.jpg

White rice, Brown Rice, Wild Rice. Staight up, basmati or "long grain" white rice is a definite high-GI food (73 GI Value) that you should avoid.

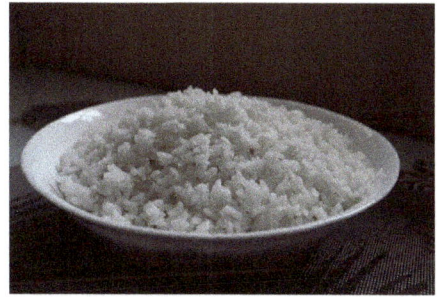

But what about "Brown Rice" or "Wile Rice". Harvard actually studied this one in their article "Brown rice versus white rice: A head-to-head comparison".[19] I can save you the article read by saying, they just aren't that different. 68 vs 73 and 241 calories vs 218 are pretty similar.

For my money, a "real" wild rice like Royal Blend's Whole Grain Wild Rice tends to come in around 45 GI. That's a whole lot better. I add some soluble fiber to a meal with it, but I love this stuff – it is just so delicious.

---

[19] See Harvard's study "Brown rice versus white rice: A head-to-head comparison"
https://www.health.harvard.edu/nutrition/brown-rice-versus-white-rice-a-head-to-head-comparison

Part III: The Soluble Fiber Solution

Chapter 6: What is Soluble Fiber?

If there's one thing you absolutely must take away from this book, it's this: You need to massively boost your soluble and dietary fiber if you want to break away from diabetes without piling on more and more medications. But what is soluble fiber? Why is it different from "regular" fiber?

Here is the definition from Wikipedia and Brittanica of soluble fiber and dietary fiber:

> **Dietary fiber or roughage** is the portion of plant-derived food that cannot be completely broken down by human digestive enzymes.[1] Dietary fibers are diverse in chemical composition, and can be grouped generally by their solubility, viscosity, and fermentability, which affect how fibers are processed in the body. Dietary fiber has two main components: soluble fiber and insoluble fiber."
> *wikipedia.org (https://en.wikipedia.org/wiki/Dietary_fiber)*

> **Soluble fibre**, which dissolves or swells in water, slows down the transit time of food through the gut (an undesirable effect) but also helps lower blood cholesterol levels (a desirable effect). Types of soluble fibre are gums, pectins, some hemicelluloses, and mucilages."
> *britannica.com (https://www.britannica.com/science/soluble-fiber)*

Soluble Fiber's Role in Controlling Blood Sugar

Here's the big difference: "regular" fiber or "dietary fiber", like you find in whole wheat bread and other so-called "healthy" foods isn't the same as soluble fiber. They are both sometimes lumped together in the term dietary fiber, but the term you really want to see and use is soluble fiber because that is the kind that will help slow the absorption of sugar in your bloodstream and keep your sugar from "spiking."

Soluble fiber basically "gums up the works" - it slows down your entire digestion process. As your body tries to digest it, this fiber turns into a thick, mushy gel that takes its sweet time moving through your system. That's exactly why it acts as a buffer against the sugar in your food

Because soluble fiber takes a long time to digest, it also makes you feel fuller, longer. This has the effect of lowering the amount of food you eat because you don't feel as hungry - which is why

> soluble fiber is the key to living life prescription-free with sugar that is controlled.

BEATING DIABETES

you lose weight when you eat this way even though you aren't even trying to portion control or "diet" in the traditional sense of the word.

As my friend Erik likes to say, "food is medicine," and soluble fiber is a wonder drug in this regard. And the fact that so much food that's rich in soluble fiber also tastes great while keeping your sugar under control is amazing. That it can let you live a "normal" life is something that should be taught in every school and every nutrition class.

And technically, it often is - but here's the problem: these powerful truths about soluble fiber get buried in wishy-washy language and half-hearted

statements. You'll see weak phrases like "can help control blood sugar" and "part of a healthy diet." Let me be crystal clear: My experience, backed by countless studies, isn't unique. Soluble fiber isn't just helpful – it's the key to living life prescription-free with well-controlled blood sugar.

As you can see in this diagram, from a 2018 article in The Atlantic[20] called **"Just Eat More Fiber"** that also quoted a 2005 study,[21] "soluble" or "dietary fiber" (they seem to be talking about the same thing) not only helps you lose weight, but it helps you regain insulin sensitivity and feeds your gut biome.

---

[20] See The Atlantic article "Just Eat More Fiber"
https://www.theatlantic.com/health/archive/2018/01/just-eat-more-fiber/550082/
[21] See the original study at Science Direct "Dietary fiber and body weight"
https://www.sciencedirect.com/science/article/abs/pii/S0899900704003041

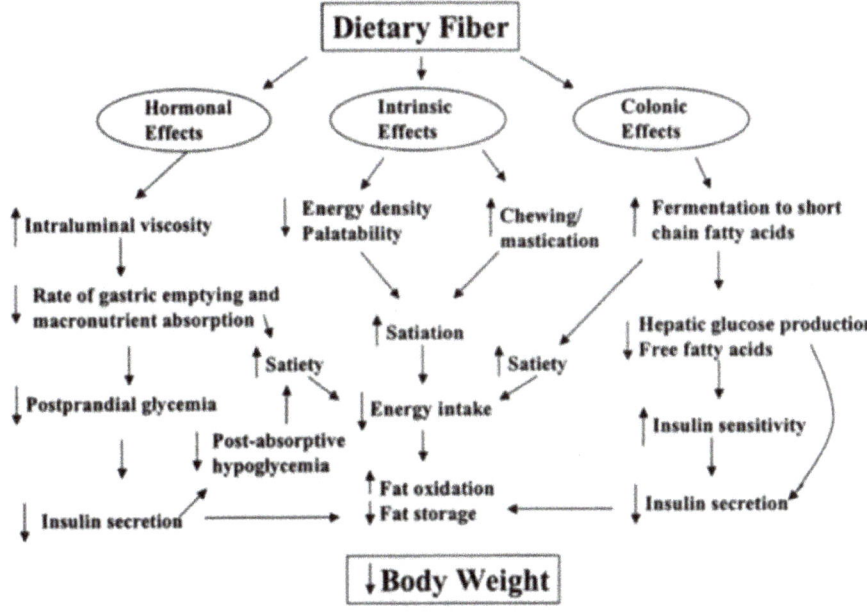

That last bit is something I think is just starting to be realized. We've known for a long time that diabetes and many other issues are either reflected in or caused by imbalances or dysfunctions of the gut. You don't have to go very far in 2025 to read articles about this phenomenon; they're on practically every Instagram, Facebook or TikTok feed.

For me, what this all says is that the "right" kinds of fiber are key to controlling not just diabetes, but many other things as well. The chart from the study mentioned above and linked to, shows that there are lots of positives, from preventing gum disease, burning fat and feeling fuller as well as less fatty acids giving you an upset stomach.

Where I disagree with this article is that its title says "Just Eat More Fiber", but the reality for diabetes remission is to **"Just Eat More Soluble Fiber."** Multigrain bread just isn't going to stop your blood sugar from going up. It is going to make it go up less than plain ole' white bread but it's going to go up a lot more than oatmeal, broccoli, edamame, hummus or any other food rich in soluble fiber.

Chapter 7: Sources of Soluble Fiber in Everyday Life

Some of my favorite foods that are both delicious and super high in soluble fiber are oatmeal (any kind that isn't loaded with added sugar), broccoli, Brussels sprouts, chickpeas and similar beans, refried beans, and lentils. Let me show you what adding these to your daily life actually looks like.

Example: White Rice vs Wild Rice

A couple of screenshots from Google searches make this crystal clear.

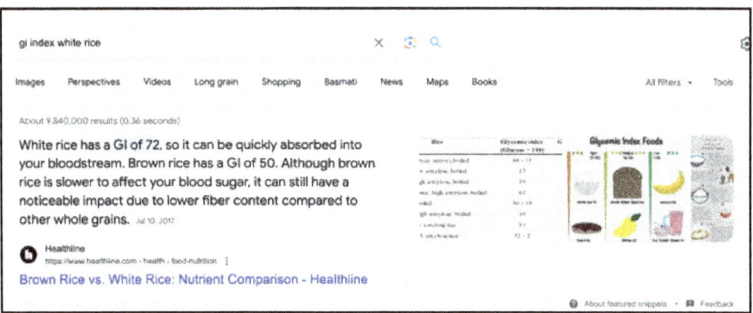

Looking at the glycemic index numbers, which we discussed previously, between white rice and wild rice, the difference jumps right out at you - wild rice comes in at just 45 on the glycemic index, while white rice hits a much higher 72.

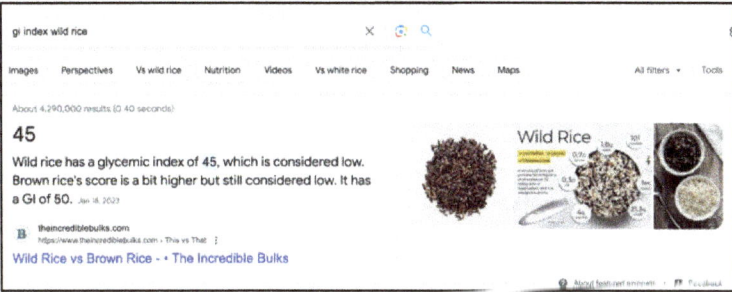

Numbers don't lie, and right here you can see exactly what I'm talking about when it comes to choosing foods that won't spike your blood sugar.

Now, most doctors say you want a GI number under 50. Looking at white rice, we're talking about a food that basically turns into glucose at high speed – that's exactly why it's a staple food worldwide. Rice gives quick energy and it's easy to grow. But if you're trying to control your sugar levels without drugs, this is one food you really need to stay away from.

Or you can load up on soluble fiber. I do both - I rarely eat white rice, but when I do, I make sure to pack in soluble fiber to help handle it. Here's a real-world example: **sushi**.

BEATING DIABETES

Sushi Example:

I love sushi. It's one of my favorite treats when going out. But here's the challenge – every roll sits on a bed of white rice. So what's a boy to do?

Check the menu at any sushi place and you'll find some "friends" that can help make this a sugar-neutral (or at least sugar-reduced) meal. My favorite helper? Edamame – young soybeans steamed and tossed with salt.

> I rarely eat white rice, but when I do, I make sure to pack in soluble fiber to help handle it.

Depending on which website you check, edamame packs 2-4 grams of soluble fiber per serving. A typical sushi restaurant portion is at least two servings, so you're getting a serious dose of soluble fiber.

So here's my strategy: I order edamame with my sushi. I usually skip the bottom layer of white rice under the fish since it doesn't add much for me (though I suppose I could just order sashimi). Once I've finished my edamame, I dig into the rolls. When I say "dig in," I'm talking about a California roll and a crunchy roll – but your mileage may vary, as they say.

The important thing to note – and you'll see this in every restaurant example in this book – is that every single menu has foods you can make work for you without anyone thinking you're "weird" or having to ask for special treatment. This is exactly what makes my approach sustainable. I never need to burden others with special requests, and I think most people feel the same way. Any "diet" that forces you to eat only-this or only-that, or demands special preparation, is a non-starter for me. Instead, I take advantage of what's already on pretty much every table and menu to control my sugar levels naturally, with almost zero fuss.

The White Foods Rule

Nutritionists have a simple rule: white foods typically turn to sugar fast in your body. White rice, white bread, potatoes, bagels – they're all bad news if you're trying to keep your sugar under control. Cauliflower is an exception to this rule and obviously oatmeal, but generally speaking you want to avoid white foods if you're looking to keep sugar under control.

This gets back to the GI Index we discussed earlier. The GI Index basically predicts how fast and completely foods convert to sugar in your body. My approach isn't about completely cutting out high-GI foods – it's about eating them sparingly and using soluble fiber strategically so I can still eat like a "normal" person.

A Word About "Whole Grains"

No offense to the whole grain enthusiasts – yes, whole grains are healthier than refined grains, and I almost always choose them over white foods. But here's the truth that might ruffle some feathers: whole grains do practically nothing for sugar control. I know that statement will get me some hate mail, but facts are facts.

Here's the reality about whole grains and insoluble fiber (what they call "roughage"): they basically pass through your digestive system intact. They don't slow digestion or help absorb sugar – so for the purpose of controlling blood sugar like I'm teaching in this book, they're just fooling you into thinking you're helping yourself.

Again, I'm not saying to avoid whole grains – they're great for your overall health. But when it comes to controlling sugar? They're just not part of the equation.

Some of the all-time greatest "hits" in the soluble fiber world

Let me share my restaurant cheat sheet: when I spot any of these items on a menu, I know I've hit the soluble fiber jackpot. Sure, you can read countless articles online about these superfoods, but what I want to emphasize is how you can find them everywhere – from steakhouses and taquerias to burger joints and fancy restaurants. Once you know what to look for, these high-soluble fiber foods are hiding in plain sight on almost every menu.

> Once you know what you're looking for, these high-soluble fiber foods are hiding in plain sight on almost every menu.

Here are my soluble fiber all-stars and where to find them:

Brussels Sprouts – 2.0 grams per serving. You'll spot these on many steakhouse menus, and they can almost balance out that baked potato you're eyeing.

Broccoli – 1.5 grams per serving and practically everywhere. Not quite as powerful as sprouts, but a reliable go-to.

Sweet Potato – I know what you're thinking – with "sweet" in the name, it must be off-limits. Actually, it packs more soluble fiber than broccoli. Just watch out for that common brown sugar topping – that'll wipe out any benefits faster than you can say "diabetes."

Beans – pretty much any kind is your friend. With 2-3 grams per serving depending on the type, they're a superfood you can't get enough of. Skip the Boston baked beans though – those kidney beans (awesome) swim in brown sugar sauce (not awesome). But here's a pro tip: at Mexican restaurants, you can "buy" your tortillas and chips with a side of refried beans.

Chickpeas (Hummus) – one of the heavyweight champs at 3 grams per serving. There's hardly a better food out there, and you're seeing it everywhere these days.

Lentils – possibly the biggest hitter of them all, packing a whopping 7-8 grams per serving! Harder to find on menus, but if you spot it, you've hit the jackpot – especially if you're planning on dessert. That Indian dal (lentils in curry)? Pure gold for your blood sugar, and absolutely delicious.

Chia Seeds – another heavy hitter (~4g/serving) that's easy to sneak into other foods without messing with taste or texture. When I see these sprinkled into yogurt or other dishes, I'm usually all in.

Fruits – Friend or Enemy and Why?

Let's talk about fruit – it's a fascinating case. On one hand, it's basically sugar (fructose). This is why so many fruit-based products are absolute no-no's for sugar control. But whole fruit itself? That's a different story – it's actually great for you, if you keep the fruit intact and avoid those refined versions.

So yes, you can absolutely enjoy fruit while controlling your sugar. In fact, a 2023 New York Times article, **"10 Nutrition Myths Experts Wish Would Die,"** tackled this head-on. They asked a straightforward question to leading nutrition experts in the United States: "What is one nutrition myth you wish would go away – and why?"

One of the myths they tackle is "Myth No. 4: People with Type 2 diabetes shouldn't eat fruit." Here's my issue with their article – while I get that they were writing for brevity, they fall into that same generic advice trap you see everywhere. They toss out statements like "And other research suggests that if you already have type 2 diabetes, eating whole fruits can help control your blood sugar" without explaining the WHY. And the why is what really matters here.

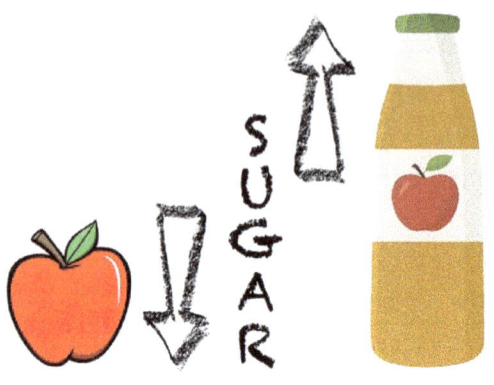

I made this diagram to illustrate the point. Apples in their "natural" state, namely with the peels and fruit intact, are just fine to eat. But when you distill them down to a juice and remove all the fruit itself and the skin and pectin and so forth, you have a high sugar product that is not good for you.

The answer, of course, comes back to our friend soluble fiber – it's in whole fruit and slows down how fast that fructose hits your system, preventing sugar spikes. So a whole apple? Good. A whole orange? Good. Blueberries? Great.

But apple juice and orange juice? They've got none of that helpful fiber because they're not the whole fruit anymore. And that blueberry compote? That's just mashed-up blueberries with a bunch of extra sugar thrown in for good measure.

> Here's the bottom line on fruit when you're controlling blood sugar: whole fruit is your friend, but all those other fruit products – juices, cocktails, fruit cups, and pretty much any other form that isn't

the actual fruit itself – are bad news and best avoided. Blueberries and apples are fantastic choices that won't mess with your sugar levels. But there's a catch with apples: keep those skins on (that's where the good stuff is) and skip the caramel dipping sauce.

Orange Juice is Enemy #1

Let me call out the biggest villain here: orange juice. I used to proudly say I was "Orange Juice Powered" – talk about an epic blunder, since I was basically main-lining sugar. But hey, I cut myself some slack on this one, since throughout the '70s and '80s we were hammered with messages about how healthy this stuff was. Here's the truth – it's not. Orange juice is basically liquid sugar with some vitamin C thrown in.

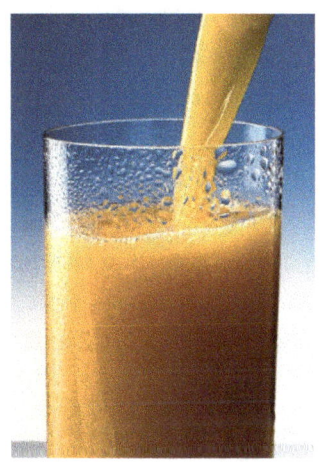

Photo credit: Wikimedia Commons[22]

Here's the deal with oranges – eat them like you did as a kid, in whole wedges. Don't squeeze out the juice and leave all that precious fiber behind.

This same principle holds true for pretty much all fruits from what I've found. Check out the glycemic index for fruits and you'll see a pattern: almost every fruit is perfectly fine if you eat it whole – skin, pulp, and all. It's when you start pulverizing, squeezing, or otherwise trying to extract the sugar while ditching the fiber that you run into trouble.

---

[22] See Wikimedia Commons "Orange juice 1 edit1"
https://commons.wikimedia.org/wiki/File:Orange_juice_1_edit1.jpg

One notable exception to this rule is the banana. There is really no meaningful fiber to slow down all that sugar. I mostly stay away from bananas, but when I do indulge, I make sure to pair it with my morning oatmeal or something similar.

How to Spot Soluble Fiber in Food

Here's a good rule of thumb: most things from the natural world – let's call them "natural foods" – are either good for sugar control or at worst neutral. Sure, you'll occasionally find exceptions like bananas that aren't great for you, but generally you can trust foods where the ingredient list is just one item. If it's just blueberries, apples, any kind of meat, or pretty much any vegetable – you're in good shape.

While we talked earlier about how cooking is chemistry, most natural foods are fine without any cooking at all. But here's something fascinating – there are some interesting exceptions where cooking actually helps. Take our old friend broccoli (one of my favorites) – it's actually better for sugar control when it's steamed than raw, coming in at 5.1 grams cooked and 2.4 grams raw.[23] Same goes for carrots. Sure, carrots are healthy either way, but cooking unlocks more of their soluble fiber. And beans? The chemistry of cooking makes them more soluble, which means better sugar control.

This all comes down to viscosity – how thick and gummy these foods get when cooked. Remember that 1978 study I mentioned in the studies section? It showed that soluble fiber helps control sugar through its viscosity. As I mentioned above, when researchers made guar gum less viscous (basically less gummy), it stopped helping insulin-resistant patients. That's some pretty powerful evidence about why cooked vegetables can work better than raw ones. That said, if I'm at a party and I want something to eat, I'm hitting up the crudité platter, having some raw broccoli and using the raw carrots to dip

---

[23] See the MyFoodData website at https://tools.myfooddata.com/nutrition-comparison/169967-170379/wt6-wt1

in the hummus. After all, I do want to have some crackers with the cheese that I love. It's all about balance.

Cinnamon

Let's talk about cinnamon – you know, that magic diabetes cure you see plastered all over TikTok and Instagram. During my journey to focusing on soluble fiber, I tried pretty much everything out there, including this one.

Here's what's out there: some studies suggest that plain old cinnamon (yes, the stuff sitting in your spice rack) might help control blood sugar, decrease insulin sensitivity, and fight diabetes. But then you've got other studies saying it does absolutely nothing. Classic case of conflicting research.

Maybe Yes

> Healthline cites an NIH study that summarizes, "Intake of 1 g of cinnamon for 12 weeks reduces fasting blood glucose and glycosylated Hb among poorly controlled type 2 diabetes patients, as well as, there is improvement in the oxidative stress markers, indicating the beneficial effect of adjuvant cinnamon as anti-diabetic and antioxidant along with conventional medications to treat poorly controlled type 2 diabetes mellitus."
>
> https://www.healthline.com/nutrition/cinnamon-and-diabetes (also https://pubmed.ncbi.nlm.nih.gov/29250843/)

Maybe No

> Another study, also from the NIH, says no discernible effect. "Results showed that using certain amount of cinnamon for 60 days did not change the glucose level of diabetic patients."
>
> https://www.ncbi.nlm.nih.gov/pmc/articles/PMC3924990/

My Own Experiment/Experience

So, I dove into all these studies – some calling it a miracle cure, others saying it was total nonsense. I thought, **"What's the harm in trying it for 12 weeks?"** I even sprung for the fancy stuff, since apparently there are two types: **Ceylon** and **Cassia**. Everything I read suggested Ceylon (the pricier one, of course) was "better"

Following the studies, I took a half teaspoon twice a day – morning and evening. Let me tell you something about half teaspoons of cinnamon: it might not sound like much, but try choking down straight cinnamon powder sometime. Instead of that warm, cozy cinnamon roll feeling you might expect, it's more like eating a packet of silica gel. The stuff completely dries out your mouth and takes real determination to get down.

After 3+ months of choking down that entire bag, my fasting levels and A1C hadn't budged. When I brought this up with my doctor, she suggested that my A1C was already too low to see any benefit.

I think she's onto something, and it might explain why the NIH ended up with two completely different results in their studies. The one showing cinnamon helped focused on "poorly controlled type-2 diabetic patients." The study showing no benefits mostly looked at housekeepers with average A1Cs of 8.9. That's not great, but I wonder if "poorly controlled" in the first study meant something even higher.

> *Bottom line: Cinnamon was a bust for me, but if you're struggling to get your A1C down, it might be worth a shot.*

A Gram is a Gram?

There's a lot of debate about how much soluble fiber it takes to 'negate' sugar from other foods. Truth is, I haven't found any scientists who've really nailed this down with solid data. The problem? Digestion has too many moving parts, and testing on real people gets messy. Instead of useful specifics, you get vague statements like this gem from the CDC: "It helps control your blood sugar and cholesterol, which can help prevent or manage diabetes complications."[24]

Nice thought, CDC, but not exactly helpful for someone trying to figure out what actually works. It's basically just a fancy way of saying "eat your vegetables like a good boy" without explaining why or how much it matters. You see these empty statements everywhere, with zero practical guidelines. As I've mentioned, it's actually one of the main reasons I wrote this book – when my friend Tim asked me how I manage my life and how he could do the same, **I couldn't point him to a single website or book that would actually help**.

For me, I use the simplest conversion possible, which is to consider one gram of soluble fiber worth one gram of sugar. I am 100% sure that there are docs and nutritionists who are going to say this is "wrong" or "not enough" or say, "it's more complicated than that."

Look, all of that is true, but let's be real – people only have so much mental bandwidth for this stuff. I want as many folks as possible to understand how soluble fiber can transform their lives, giving them control over diabetes and even the power to reverse it. That means giving people simple rules they can actually use.

> **I USE THE SIMPLEST CONVERSION POSSIBLE, WHICH IS TO CONSIDER ONE GRAM OF SOLUBLE FIBER WORTH ONE GRAM OF ADDED SUGAR.**

---

[24] See the CDC website "Fiber: The Carb That Helps You Manage Diabetes" https://www.cdc.gov/diabetes/healthy-eating/fiber-helps-diabetes.html

In Chapter 11, we'll walk through tons of real-world food examples and how I decide what to eat. I go through several real menus and food labels in stores so you can see how I view these things and figure out what to eat.

I'll be using this "rule" as I go through those examples, even though I know it's probably not perfect science.

Here's why I do these calculations of sugar grams this way: I'm a regular adult with a family and work I need to show up for – I need simple rules to help me live my life, and I bet most of you do too. My apologies to the doctors and nutritionists for my oversimplifying things, but this is how I roll with it. And you know what? It works for me and for others I've shared it with.

Chapter 8: Studies I Bet My Life On

It was a challenge to research this book. I had to read a bunch of studies that oftentimes went over my head. Additionally, in the United States we don't really work on reversing or controlling diabetes much, so you're often reading materials from other countries or studies that almost, but not exactly, are what you need them to be about or where the conclusions are intriguing but no follow up was made.

Here are some of the key studies and articles that really helped me out in my quest to understand how to control sugar. This is not an exhaustive list, and it is growing all the time. This is because so many people are diagnosed with Diabetes Type 2 that researchers are really focusing on studying the root causes. This is causing the tide to somewhat turn in the medical establishment and making it acceptable to believe that lifestyle changes can be done effectively and that they will work if the patient sticks to them.

Newcastle University (UK) - The power of soluble fiber to control blood sugar metabolization and "reverse" diabetes[25]

This is a landmark study that showed that diabetes can be reversed and that fat on the pancreas is the extant cause. Based on work in 2008 and 2011 it shows that Type 2 Diabetes has specific causes that can be understood and that there are non-medical ways in which this could be controlled. To say this was the most important thing I learned is an understatement.

I quote some of the relevant quotes from the study here:

- "Type 2 diabetes is caused by a small amount of excess fat inside the liver and inside the pancreas"

- "It is a potentially reversible condition"

- If a person has type 2 diabetes, they have become too heavy for their own body (nothing to do with the arbitrary concept of obesity)

- Weight loss of around 15kg is necessary for most people to reverse diabetes or to put it into remission

- People with type 2 diabetes but have a "normal" body mass index have an excess of hidden fat and should aim to lose around 10% of body weight

---

[25] See Reversing Type 2 Diabetes and ongoing remission
https://www.ncl.ac.uk/magres/research/diabetes/reversal/#publicinformation

BEATING DIABETES

- This can be achieved using a simple 3-step method: the 1, 2, 3 of diabetes reversal

- Type 2 diabetes is most easily reversed to normal in the early years after diagnosis

- "How and why type 2 diabetes happens can now be understood"

There's even a Guardian article on a guy who had a very similar experience to myself[26].

Diabetes (UK) – The DiRECT study[27]

The DiRECT study was created "To determine whether a structured weight management programme, delivered in a realistic Primary Care setting, is a viable treatment for producing T2DM remission. Extend current knowledge about the mechanisms behind T2DM and its remission."

> https://www.diabetes.org.uk/about-us/news-and-views/weight-loss-can-put-type-2-diabetes-remission-least-five-years-reveal-latest-findings

This is an update from the DiRECT study for 2024. In it they indicate that my experience with soluble fiber is both replicable and long-lasting. The DiRECT Study is one of the first ones I read about where the idea that one could push diabetes into remission or even eliminate it was put forward and tested.

NIH (US)

Dietary fibres, fibre analogues, and glucose tolerance: importance of viscosity.
https://www.ncbi.nlm.nih.gov/pmc/articles/PMC1604761/

---

[26] See "Type 2 diabetes and the diet that cured me"
https://www.theguardian.com/lifeandstyle/2013/may/12/type-2-diabetes-diet-cure
[27] See the Study's website "Diabetes Remission Clinical Trial"
https://www.directclinicaltrial.org.uk/

A landmark study from way back in 1978 showed that viscosity of foods affects blood sugar in a material way. It is this study that provided the first serious underpinnings on understanding that soluble fiber is the key way to control blood sugar for insulin sensitive people and diabetics. It is also one of the places I got the idea to look for remission or removal of diabetes as a possibility.

Effects of dietary fiber and carbohydrate on glucose and lipoprotein metabolism in diabetic patients
https://pubmed.ncbi.nlm.nih.gov/1663443/

There are two very relevant quotes from this one, titled "Effects of dietary fiber and carbohydrate on glucose and lipoprotein metabolism in diabetic patients."

> *"It has been shown repeatedly that a high-carbohydrate diet increases plasma insulin and triglyceride levels and can deteriorate blood glucose control in the postprandial period. However, much of the controversy between advocates and detractors of dietary carbohydrate can be settled by taking into account dietary fiber."*

> *"A balanced increase in consumption of fiber-rich foods and unsaturated fat is the most rational way to replace foods rich in saturated fat and cholesterol in the diabetic diet."*

What is interesting here is that they get to the same data points but ignore the conclusion that soluble fiber is the strongest lever you have to help you control and even eliminate diabetes. This sort of prevarication is why I say that the U.S. medical establishment is not on board with anything other than the idea that diabetes is uncurable and only the symptoms can be treated.

What is frustrating is that other NIH studies[28] show the effects, but their conclusions, which would help spread the word to the people who need to hear it, go unnoticed.

Nutrition Journal[29]

This is a randomized control trial from 2016 where the participants were overweight (mean BMI >31) and were given a diet rich in soluble fiber. This showed a very notable change in both weight as well as sugar control.

> "After 8 weeks of intervention, soluble fiber supplementation showed significant reduction in the intervention group in BMI ($p < 0.001$) when compared with the control group. Moreover, water soluble fiber supplementation proven to improve FBS (163 to 119 mg/dl), HbA1C (8.5 to 7.5 %), insulin level (27.9 to 19.7 µIU/mL), C-peptide (5.8 to 3.8 ng/ml), HOMA.IR (11.3 to 5.8) and HOMA-β % (103 to 141 %)."

Compare this to my experience where I really jacked up soluble carbs, especially when I was first fighting to get my sugar under control. In their study, eight weeks was enough to go from 8.5 to 7.5 – I did roughly 3.5-4 points in just about the same period.

So, in 2016, we have serious studies that support the idea that soluble fiber can literally remove medication from patients' lives and almost no medical professional I have ever asked has heard about what this showed. Or they say things like "fiber is an important part of a healthy diet" without the emphasis that it can literally change your medical outcomes.

---

[28] See NIH article – "The Effects of Soluble Dietary Fibers on Glycemic Response: An Overview and Futures Perspectives"
https://www.ncbi.nlm.nih.gov/pmc/articles/PMC9736284/

[29] See article from Biomedical Central – "Soluble fibers from psyllium improve glycemic response and body weight among diabetes type 2 patients (randomized control trial)"
https://nutritionj.biomedcentral.com/articles/10.1186/s12937-016-0207-4

Harvard[30]

What I really love about this article is that it describes fiber in detail and the different ways in which we can think and talk about it.

"Further defining fiber

>Under the umbrella terms of insoluble and soluble fibers, you may see fiber described in other ways. It can be *viscous* with a gel-like quality, or *fermentable* because it acts as food for gut bacteria that breaks it down and ferments it. Fibers that are not broken down by bacteria, called *nonfermentable*, travel intact to the colon and can add bulk and weight to stool so it is easier to pass. These properties offer health benefits such as slowing down digestion, delaying blood sugar rises after meals, promoting healthy colonies of bacteria, or having a laxative effect. In addition, there are many subtypes of soluble and insoluble fibers, some of which occur naturally in plant foods and others that are synthetically made.

"Naturally occurring plant fibers:

- *Cellulose* – Insoluble fiber found in cereal grains and the cell walls of many fruits and vegetables. It absorbs water and adds bulk to stool, which can have a laxative effect.
- *Lignins* – Insoluble fiber found in wheat and corn bran, nuts, flaxseeds, vegetables, and unripe bananas that triggers mucus secretion in the colon and adds bulk to stools. Has laxative effect.
- *Beta-glucans* – Soluble highly fermentable fiber found in oats and barley that is metabolized and fermented in the small intestine. Acts as a prebiotic. Can add bulk to stool but does not have a laxative effect. May help to normalize blood glucose and cholesterol levels.
- *Guar gum* – Soluble fermentable fiber isolated from seeds. Has a viscous gel texture and is often added to foods as a thickener. It is metabolized and fermented in the small intestine. Does not have a

---

[30] See Harvard "Fiber" Study info at
https://www.hsph.harvard.edu/nutritionsource/carbohydrates/fiber/

laxative effect. May help to normalize blood sugar and cholesterol levels.
- *Inulin* – Soluble fermentable fibers found in onions, chicory root, asparagus, and Jerusalem artichokes. May help to bulk stool with a laxative effect, normalize blood glucose, and act as a prebiotic. People with irritable bowel syndrome may be sensitive to these fibers that can cause bloating or stomach upset.
- *Pectins* – Soluble highly fermentable fiber found in apples, berries, and other fruits. Minimal bulking or laxative effect. Due to its gelling properties, it may slow digestion and help normalize blood sugar and cholesterol levels.
- *Resistant starch* – Soluble fermentable fiber found in legumes, unripe bananas, cooked and cooled pasta, and potatoes that acts as a prebiotic. Adds bulk to stools but has minimal laxative effect. May help to normalize blood sugar and cholesterol levels.

Manufactured fibers, some of which are extracted and modified from natural plants:

- *Psyllium* – Soluble viscous nonfermentable fiber extracted from psyllium seeds that holds onto water and softens and bulks stools. Has laxative effect and is an ingredient in over-the-counter laxatives and high-fiber cereals. May help to normalize blood sugar and cholesterol levels.
- *Polydextrose and polyols* – Soluble fiber made of glucose and sorbitol, a sugar alcohol. It can increase stool bulk and have a mild laxative effect. Minimal effect on blood sugar or cholesterol levels. It is a food additive used as a sweetener, to improve texture, maintain moisture, or to increase fiber content.
- *Inulin, oligosaccharides, pectins, resistant starch, gums* – Soluble fibers derived from plant foods as listed above, but are isolated or modified into a concentrated form that is added to foods or fiber supplements."

While this list of descriptions is a bit on the technical side, if you read through it you can start seeing what to eat pretty clearly. This was one of my major sources of understanding early on.

CDC (US)[31]

This article has a great title – "***Fiber: The Carb That Helps You Manage Diabetes***". While the rest of the article is not as clear as one could hope for, it does lay out the basic issues pretty clearly. My favorite quote from this is "Here's the scoop. Fiber is a type of carbohydrate found mainly in fruits, vegetables, whole grains, and legumes. It helps keep you regular, but it offers many other health benefits as well, especially for people with diabetes or prediabetes."

Can't put things clearer than that – but this is also a site that tells you things like "Diabetes is a chronic (long-lasting) health condition that affects how your body turns food into energy." While true, this is the kind of article where you might mention to people that there's actual studied outcomes where this "chronic" condition can be pushed out of people's lives – effectively eliminated.

Yet it is in a 2012 CDC study[32] where they show that "The ILI group (the ones with lifestyle/food changes) was significantly more likely to experience any remission (partial or complete)." It's 2025 and so frustrating that we still can't be clear with people that diabetes is not incurable, and it can be put in remission.

Health Castle

> "An average diet contains 1:3 soluble fiber to insoluble fiber ratio. In a small study published in 2017, UC Davis researchers compared the difference of 3:1 soluble to insoluble fiber ratio versus a 1:3 ratio. They tested on satiety, glucose response, insulin response, and more. Results showed that 3:1 soluble to insoluble fiber diet significantly increased satiety and decreased hunger. In addition, insulin response was the lowest in the 3:1 soluble to insoluble group. In other words,

---

[31] See the CDC Fiber: The Carb That Helps You Manage Diabetes
https://www.cdc.gov/diabetes/library/features/role-of-fiber.html

[32] See Association of an Intensive Lifestyle Intervention With Remission of Type 2 Diabetes
https://stacks.cdc.gov/view/cdc/38316

the body responded to the diet with secreting less insulin, suggesting that insulin sensitivity may have been improved. This result suggested that a greater proportion of soluble fiber may have better metabolic benefits."

https://www.healthcastle.com/fiber-101-soluble-fiber-vs-insoluble-fiber/

And

https://nutrition.ucdavis.edu/outreach/nutr-health-info-sheets/inulin

Further Research

There are many, many studies on these issues and I encourage everyone who wants to control their sugar and either reverse or put diabetes into remission to become a good student of them. This is an evolving area of human knowledge, and more information is gained constantly.

While it is true that type 2 diabetes is a progressive disease that can be controlled with drugs, that is _not_ the final word. That is only true if it is left untreated or without food-based interventions of the sort I have written about in this book.

I am not Superman, and I do not have a whole lot of self-control or discipline. However, using these techniques I never even got a second high A1C reading. _**I took control of my sugar using**_

> My methods for living a "normal" life without prescription drugs to control diabetes are within the reach of most people. I dropped my A1C from super-high to elevated to normal to low in under six months. I do not think I'm special or an outlier.

well-researched methods backed by studies that you can read on your own.

My methods for living a "normal" life without prescription drugs to control diabetes are within the reach of most people.

I dropped my A1C from super-high to elevated to normal to low in under six months. I do not think I'm special or an outlier.

What I do think is that very few people who are diagnosed diabetic or have a high A1C reading have heard about an option that doesn't start with a prescription. I think that their doctors tell them what my first post-A1C explosion doctor said – here's some meds, you're going to need a whole lot more because this is progressive and incurable. It's the easy button for overworked primary care physicians who also hear "I'm going to change my lifestyle" too many times.

I'm pretty sure people think they need to diet – that they need to take a magic pill like Ozempic. But what is proven to be within their reach and is shown to be effective is to up their intake of soluble fiber and lower their sugar and sugar-metabolizing carbs as much as possible.

This is not particularly hard to do, and it doesn't limit you from going to a restaurant or force you to cook special meals. It just takes education and training to know what to eat and what to avoid and how to read a nutrition label.

When you look at the foods in the next chapter on labels, they aren't any more expensive than "regular" foods. They're actually in many cases cheaper. It takes a bit more thought and learning – but that beats the hell out of shooting yourself up twice a day with insulin for the rest of your life while changing a Dexcom every ten days.

Part IV: Practical Implementation

Chapter 9: Reading Nutrition Labels for Sugar Control

If you're trying to control your sugar, you've got to learn to read nutritional labels like a detective. Why? Because food companies and marketers are playing fast and loose with what they call 'healthy.'

Here's the simple version: **Look for foods where the soluble fiber number is higher than the added sugar number.**

We've talked about how soluble fiber is your best friend for sugar control, and how the glycemic index can help guide your food choices. But let's get real – most of your food comes from a store, in packages with those government-required nutrition labels.

Thank goodness for the activists who've pushed the FDA to keep improving these labels over the years. While the labels are always changing, right now they mostly tell you what you need to know to make smart choices. After all, soluble fiber might be your sugar-fighting superhero, but that doesn't help much if you can't spot it at the grocery store.

> Look for foods where the soluble fiber number is higher than the added sugar number.

Get ready for a tour through the grocery store aisles, where I'm going to call out some brands that market themselves as *healthy* – and sure, maybe they are for some people, but not if you're trying to control your sugar. I'll probably catch some heat for this (or get "'hated on'" as my daughter would say), but I think you need real examples of real brands to make informed decisions.

Listen, I've eaten my share of junk food over the years – and man, do I love a poppyseed bagel – but that stuff doesn't work for me anymore. I need to spot the right foods quickly and easily, especially when I'm traveling and can't get my usual stuff. So, with apologies to the brands I'm about to use as examples, here's what I look for when reading a food label.

The golden rule of sugar control: *get your soluble fiber level higher than your sugar intake*. When you hit this sweet spot (pun intended), you kick off a virtuous cycle that helps control insulin resistance and delivers all the other benefits we've been talking about in this book.

BEATING DIABETES

But here's the thing – you can't do this if you don't know what's in your food or how to decode those nutrition labels. So, in this chapter, we're going to walk through real-life examples that will give you the practical tools to make this work.

A Gram, A Teaspoon and A Sugar Packet

Here's a reality check: Like most Americans, I haven't got a clue what a gram looks like. Yet somehow every food label uses grams. I'm sure there's a good reason for this, but my cynical side says it's just another way to keep Americans confused about what's actually in their food.

But there's no getting around it – almost everything on these labels uses metric measurements that most of us in the United States just can't process instinctively.

> A teaspoon of sugar is about 4-4.5 grams. Just call it 4 because the math is easy.

To understand this in sugar terms we can use the following conversions:

A teaspoon of sugar is about 4-4.5 grams. Just call it 4 because the math is easy.

Depending on whether you check Quora, the NHS, Omni Calculator, or just Google it, you'll get answers ranging from a super-precise 4.16667 to "about 4.8 grams" per teaspoon. Here's what I do: I just round it to 4 grams per teaspoon and divide by four. Why teaspoons? Because that's what most of us, including me, actually use when we're putting sugar in our coffee or on our cereal.

> A sugar packet is 3.5 grams of sugar, or slightly less than a teaspoon.

A sugar packet is 3.5 grams of sugar, or slightly less than a teaspoon.

I use Domino sugar packets as my reference point – they're like the Kleenex™ of sugar packets. Sure, there are hundreds of competitors, but Domino is the one everyone knows. Right on their website, they tell us "Conveniently enjoy every sweet moment with Domino® Sugar Packets. Each packet contains 3.5 grams of pure cane sugar."

Example: Yogurt

Let's put this conversion to work with something almost everyone's eaten – yogurt. I'm going to show you two labels: Chobani Plain Yogurt and Chobani Blueberry Yogurt. I'm using these because they're everywhere – grocery stores, convenience stores, hotel breakfast bars, you name it.

When you're looking to control sugar, here's a shortcut: zoom in on just the carbs section of the nutrition label. That's where you'll find our friends dietary fiber, fiber, and soluble fiber. Sometimes they break these out nicely for us, but often (for reasons I can't fathom) they don't.

The key thing to note in those two products is **that the plain yogurt has 0 grams added sugar and blueberry has 9 grams**.

> Zoom in on just the carbs section of the nutrition label. That's where you'll find our friends and enemies…

BEATING DIABETES

NUTRITION FACTS		
Serving size 1 container (150g)		
Amount Per Serving		
Calories		**110**
		% Daily Value*
Total Fat 0g		0%
Saturated Fat 0g		0%
Trans Fat 0g		
Cholesterol 5mg		2%
Sodium 55mg		2%
Total Carbohydrates 16g		6%
Fiber <1g		3%
Total Sugars 14g		
Including 9g Added Sugars		18%
Protein 11g		22%
Vitamin D 0%	Potassium	4%
Iron 0%	Calcium	10%

*The % Daily Value (DV) tells you how much a nutrient in a serving of food contributes to a daily diet. 2,000 calories a day is used for general nutrition advice.

BLUEBERRY YOGURT

Nutrition Facts		
About 5 servings per container		
Serving size		3/4 cup (170g)
Amount per serving		
Calories		**90**
		% Daily Value*
Total Fat 0g		0%
Saturated Fat 0g		0%
Trans Fat 0g		
Cholesterol 10mg		3%
Sodium 65mg		3%
Total Carbohydrate 6g		2%
Dietary Fiber 0g		0%
Total Sugars 4g		
Incl. 0g Added Sugars		0%
Protein 16g		32%
Vit. D 0mcg 0% • Calcium 187mg 15%		
Iron 0mg 0% • Potas. 250mg 6%		

*The % Daily Value (DV) tells you how much a nutrient in a serving of food contributes to a daily diet. 2,000 calories a day is used for general nutrition advice.

PLAIN YOGURT

Plain Yogurt's got its natural sugars, and whole blueberries are balanced – we looked at this in Chapter 7 (Sources of Soluble Fiber in Everyday Life). **But look at this "blueberry yogurt" – it's packing two heaping teaspoons of sugar, almost three full sugar packets!** The problem isn't the natural sugar from the blueberries – it's all that extra sugar they've dumped in there!

Sure, our conversion method isn't perfect science, but it gives you a quick, easy way to spot how much sugar – especially that sneaky added sugar – is lurking in your food.

The Carb Section

As you've seen from our yogurt example, when you're checking for sugar control, you really only need to look at one part of the label: the carbohydrates section. This is your gold mine – it shows both the natural sugars (like from whole fruit) and any sugar they've added to the product.

> **For sugar control, the only part of the nutrition label you need to pay attention to is the carbs section.**

These are your detective tools in the nutrition label: the fiber content (both type and amount), total sugar, and that crucial added sugar number.

Armed with these data points, we can pull back the curtain and see who's really pulling a fast one in the Land of Oz (okay, I know – that was a seriously mixed metaphor!). But here's the truth: these four or five lines are all you need to decide if a food works for your sugar control.

Cereal

Let's hit the cereal aisle – and brace yourself, because in my experience, there's barely a truly healthy cereal to be found. Most of those so-called "healthy" choices? They're loaded with added sugar and terrible for sugar control.

But here's the thing: I love cereal. So I had to figure out what I could actually eat from that aisle. Let's start with some classics – **Rice Krispies, Cheerios, Wheaties, Special K, and Frosted Mini-Wheats**. I'm not even going to waste time on Cocoa Puffs or Captain Crunch – if you're reading this book and don't already know to avoid those, we need to have a different conversation.

We'll also look at some cereals that market themselves as "healthy" and break down which ones actually work for sugar control and which ones are disasters. I'm talking about **Grape Nuts**, **Kashi Go Crunch**, and **Purely Elizabeth Honey Peanut Butter Superfood**.

Here's the surprising thing you'll discover: there's often a huge gap between what you expect to be good for you and what actually is. Those nutrition labels are your reality check for making choices that support your goals. This is why the BBC wrote an article recently called "Are breakfast cereals really good for us?"[33]

Don't get fooled by all those "whole grains" and "great source of fiber" claims plastered all over the cereal aisle. Remember what we learned earlier – whole grains might be healthy, but they don't do much for sugar control. They're not going to offset that "added sugar" number one bit.

---

[33] See "Are breakfast cereals really good for us?" at https://www.bbc.com/future/article/20250422-are-breakfast-cereals-really-good-for-us

Cheerios

This is one of the best cereals out there. Not only does it taste good, but it's about the only one you'll find where the soluble fiber and sugar are actually in balance.

I basically stick to three cereals: regular Cheerios (not Honey Nut or any of those other varieties), Wheaties, or Total. And yes, I do add a tiny bit of sugar to my Cheerios – we're talking a quarter teaspoon in a whole bowl. Just enough to give it a little flavor boost, but not enough to cause trouble.

Nutrition Facts

Serving size: 1 1/2 cup (39g) (age 4+ years)

Amount per serving
Calories **140**
As Packaged

Food component / Nutrient	Amount As Packaged	% DV* As Packaged
Total Fat	2.5g	3%
Saturated Fat	0.5g	3%
Trans Fat	0g	—
Polyunsaturated Fat	1g	—
Monounsaturated Fat	1g	—
Cholesterol	0mg	0%
Sodium	190mg	8%
Total Carbohydrate	29g	10%
Dietary Fiber	4g	15%
Soluble Fiber	2g	—
Total Sugars	2g	—
Incl. Added Sugars	1g	2%
Protein	5g	—
Vitamin D	4mcg	20%

Example: Kashi Go Crunch

Here's another one of those "health food" cereals. Sure, it" got a decent amount of Dietary Fiber, though they don't tell us how much is soluble.

But even if every bit of that fiber was soluble, this is still a sugar bomb. You're looking at 5 grams more sugar than fiber, <u>13 grams total</u>. Let me put that in perspective – **it's like dumping 3 heaping spoonfuls of sugar or emptying 4 sugar packets into your bowl!**

Nutrition Facts

Serving Size 53 G
Servings Per Container 7

Amount Per Serving	
Calories	190
Calories From Fat	25
	% Daily Value
Total Fat 3 G	5
Saturated Fat 0 G	0
Trans Fat 0 G	
Cholesterol 0 Mg	0
Sodium 105 Mg	4
Potassium 290 Mg	8
Total Carboydrate 39 G	13
Dietary Fiber 8 G	32
Sugars 13 G	
Protein 8 G	
Vitamin A	0
Vitamin C	0
Calcium	4
Phosphorus	15
Magnesium	10

Look, I get it – I used to do that kind of thing in college when I was 19 or 20. But if you're trying to control your sugar, you need to stay away from this stuff, no matter how many times they put "health food" on the box.

Example: Purely Elizabeth Honey Peanut Butter Superfood

I guess I shouldn't be shocked, but this one actually made "Women's Health's list of 10 healthiest cereals in 2023".Shows you just how misleading those lists can be. Let's look at what the label actually tells us.

You can see there's a decent amount of Dietary Fiber (4 grams). They don't break it out, but I suspect a lot of it is whole fiber rather than soluble fiber. But hey, let's be generous and pretend it's all soluble fiber.

Even then, with 7g of added sugar (that's basically two sugar packets) in every bowl, this is way over our target. Remember our golden rule for everything we're discussing in this chapter: **your soluble fiber number should be greater than or equal to your added sugars.** As we covered earlier, 'natural' sugars like those in whole blueberries are fine – it's the blueberry compote or jam you need to watch out for. Whole or cut-up fruit is natural sugar (more on that in Chapter 6).

But looking at Elizabeth's "Superfood" here, we're seeing 3 grams more added sugar per serving than fiber. So despite the fancy marketing, this one's a no-go.

Example: Grape Nuts

While some people don't like the taste, and others might find it tough on their teeth, this stuff isn't bad. Not as good as regular Cheerios – but hey, not many things are.

Notice how they separate dietary fiber from soluble fiber and claim no added sugars. But here's what makes me suspicious: 5 grams of total sugar in a product with no fruit? Something's not adding up. Makes me think there's some sneaky added sugar hiding in there somewhere.

Sure, Grape Nuts is way better than turning your blood sugar into a roller coaster with Captain Crunch. But with those mystery sugars, I'd probably still give this one a pass.

"Granola" Bars or "Nutrition" Bars

Nature's Bakery – Blueberry... "Almost as good as Oreos"

From 2017 to 2019, I was convinced these things were the bomb. They were delicious, and I thought they were good for me. I even stocked my office with them and packed three boxes for a trip through northern India. But

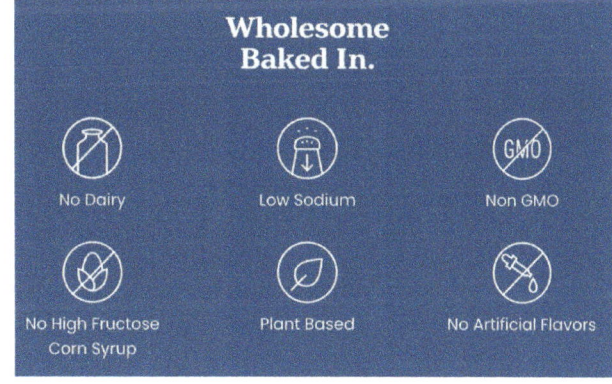

once I understood the power of soluble fiber and how crucial the balance between fiber and sugar really is, I realized I'd been fooling myself.

BEATING DIABETES

Let's look at their marketing: "No High Fructose Corn Syrup," "Plant based," "No Artificial Flavors" – this is straight from their website in 2024, and it hasn't changed much over the years. But check this out: 14g of Added Sugars!!! That's about **4 sugar packets added per package**! **Literally the same as a package of three Oreos.**

Here's the thing – no offense to Nature's Bakery, but if I'm going to have that much added sugar, I"d rather just eat the Oreos. At least Oreos are honest about what they are. They're delicious cookies that might be the greatest thing ever dunked in milk, but they're not pretending to be health food.

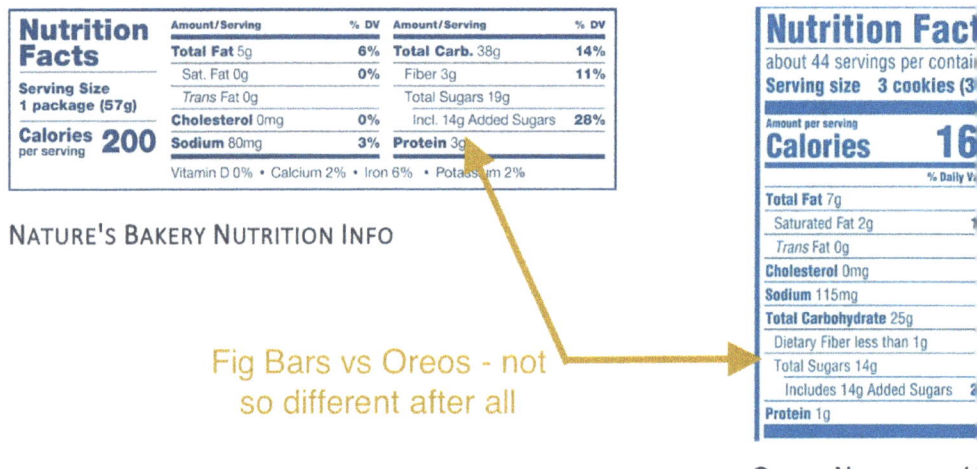

NATURE'S BAKERY NUTRITION INFO

Fig Bars vs Oreos - not so different after all

OREOS NUTRITION INFO

This kind of deceptive labeling is everywhere, which shows just how crucial those FDA-required labels with real numbers are. And listen – I consider myself pretty savvy when it comes to reading labels, but this one had me fooled for two whole years before I finally caught on.

BEATING DIABETES

Kind – some Kinds of Kind are Kinder Than Others

Here's something that might surprise you: even within the same brand, some products are great for sugar control while others are disasters.

Take Cheerios – the range goes from awesome to awful depending on which box you grab. Original Cheerios? A winner. But those fancy flavored versions? Not so much. Kind bars are the perfect example of this – some of their products are decent choices, others are sugar bombs. This is exactly why reading labels matters so much. Let's look at two of their bars, for instance.

CARAMEL & SEA SALT

Nutrition Facts		
Serving Size	1 bar (40g)	
	Amount / Serving	% Daily Value
Calories	170	
Total Fat	15g	19%
Saturated Fat	3g	15%
Trans Fat	0g	
Polyunsaturated Fat	3.5g	
Monounsaturated Fat	9g	
Cholesterol	0mg	0%
Sodium	125mg	5%
Total Carbohydrate	16g	6%
Dietary Fiber	7g	25%
Total Sugars	5g	
Includes 4g Added Sugars		8%
Sugar Alcohol	0g	
Protein	6g	
Vitamin D		0%
Calcium		6%
Iron		6%
Potassium		4%

DARK CHOCOLATE, PEANUT BUTTER, ALMOND

Nutrition Facts		
Serving Size	1 bar (40g)	
	Amount / Serving	% Daily Value
Calories	200	
Total Fat	14g	18%
Saturated Fat	4g	20%
Trans Fat	0g	
Polyunsaturated Fat	2.5g	
Monounsaturated Fat	6g	
Cholesterol	0mg	0%
Sodium	20mg	1%
Total Carbohydrate	17g	6%
Dietary Fiber	3g	11%
Total Sugars	9g	
Includes 8g Added Sugars		16%
Sugar Alcohol	0g	
Protein	7g	
Vitamin D		0%
Calcium		2%
Iron		6%
Potassium		4%

You'd probably think that since both have something sweet in the name (Caramel and Dark Chocolate), they'd be pretty similar sugar-wise. But lets see what the labels tell us...

Here's the surprise: the Caramel bar is actually much better for sugar control, with 2 more grams of Dietary Fiber than added sugar (though I wish they'd break down how much is soluble). The Dark Chocolate version? Not so kind to your blood sugar – just 3 grams of fiber but a whopping 8 grams of added sugar!

BEATING DIABETES

Would it be better to snack on hummus and carrots? Of course. But if you need a shelf-stable snack that won't send your sugar through the roof, go for the Caramel bar and skip that Dark Chocolate and Peanut Butter one.

Chapter 10: Recipes that kick A$$ For Soluble Fiber

Let's get real here: yes, you need to boost your soluble fiber, and sure, broccoli and Brussels sprouts are great. But nobody wants to live on vegetables alone. Food should bring joy to life – after all, the whole point of getting off the drugs and controlling sugar is to live well, not just exist.

So let me share some recipes that actually taste amazing while delivering that soluble fiber punch. These are family favorites – some from my beloved wife, some from me – that prove healthy eating doesn't have to be boring.

Baked Breakfast Oatmeal

I live for this stuff – it's my go-to breakfast every single day, mixed with some yogurt. Not only is it delicious and keeps me full, but it's also loaded with soluble fiber and barely any sugar. The best part? My wife, Kendra, keeps it interesting by changing it up based on whatever fruit we've got on hand. Sometimes she'll throw in some cut apples, other times strawberries, and there are almost always blueberries in there – often it's a mix of whatever looks good.

Kendra's Baked Oatmeal

Cook Time: 35-40 minutes Servings: Servings: 12-14

Source: Originally Epicurious.com but Kendra has altered it quite a bit.
Photo credit: Christopher Reade

Ingredients

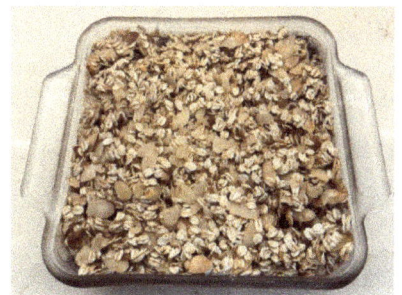

- 2 or 3 very ripe or frozen bananas
- Your choice of fruit
- One egg
- Vanilla
- Cinnamon
- Oats (rolled or steel cut)
- Milk (2% or Whole)
- Salt

Directions

Heat oven to 375°F

Start by mashing three ripe bananas into an even layer in an 8x8 pan. Pro tip: use frozen-then-thawed bananas – they work best.

Add your fruit layer. This is where it gets fun – you can use fresh berries, frozen berries, apple chunks with raisins or cranberries, figs... whatever you've got around!

In a separate bowl:

- Beat one egg
- Add 1 tsp vanilla
- 1/2 tsp cinnamon
- 1/2 tsp salt
- 2 cups rolled oats (not quick or instant – this matters!)
- 2 cups milk
- 1 cup sliced almonds

Mix it all up and pour over your fruit layer. Bake for 35-40 minutes.

The beauty of this recipe? Cover it well and it'll last all week in the fridge. Just zap a serving for 30 seconds in the microwave when you want it. I love mine with a dollop of yogurt on top, but that's totally optional.

Baked Feta with Tomatoes and Chickpeas

Cook Time: 35 minutes Servings:
Servings: 4
Source: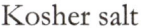
Photo: Wikimedia Commons[34]

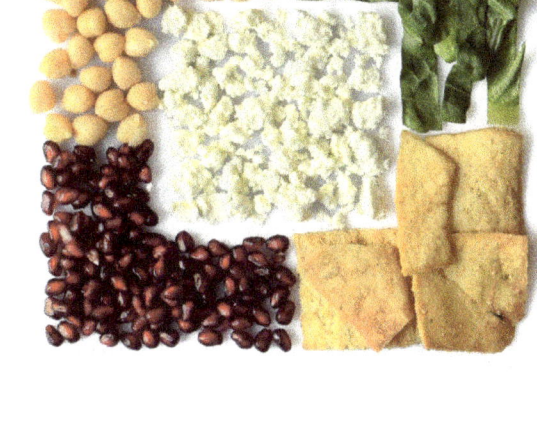

Ingredients

8-ounce (225-gram) block feta
1/2 cup (120 ml) olive oil
1 1/2 to 2 pints (3 to 4 cups) cherry or grape tomatoes
4 garlic cloves, thinly sliced
1/2 a red chili pepper, thinly sliced
Kosher salt
Freshly ground black pepper
2 (15-ounce) cans chickpeas, drained and rinsed
2 to 3 tablespoons fresh chopped herbs (parsley, cilantro, mint, dill, basil, or rosemary, or a mix)
Flatbread or toasted pita wedges (gluten-free, if needed), for serving

Directions

Heat your oven to 400°F.

---

[34] See Wikimedia Commons
https://commons.wikimedia.org/wiki/File:Chickpea_lettuce_salad_garbanzo_beans_(28151568544).jpg

Place a block of feta in the middle of a 9×13-inch (or any 3-quart) baking dish. Drizzle olive oil over and around it. Add tomatoes to the oil-coated pan, then sprinkle them with:

- Minced garlic
- 1/2 teaspoon kosher salt
- A few good grinds of black pepper

Toss to coat everything in oil, then scatter some chili pepper over the feta.

Now for the timing:

1. First round: Roast 15 minutes, until the tomatoes start getting juicy
2. Add the chickpeas around the feta, plus another hit of salt and pepper. Stir to coat with oil
3. Back in the oven for 10 more minutes (or until tomatoes reach your preferred juiciness)
4. Final step: Switch to broiler (or crank the heat as high as it'll go) for 5-8 minutes until the tomatoes and feta get some nice color

For serving, you've got options: either stir that melty feta into the tomato-chickpea mixture, or do what I do and leave it in the center, scooping some with each serving. Finish with a scatter of fresh herbs.

Chocolate Chia Pudding

Prep Time: 5 mins

Cook Time: 0 mins

Servings: Servings 2 servings

Source: feelgoodfoodie.net plus Kendra's edits

Photo Credit: WikiMedia Commons[35]

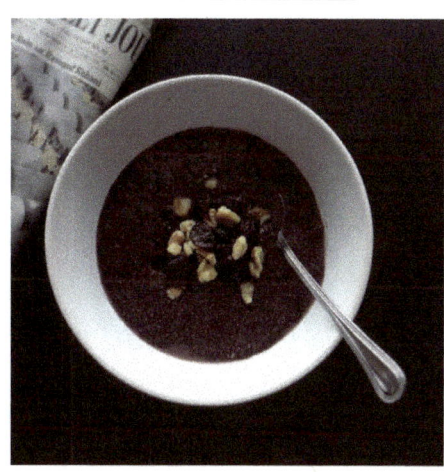

Ingredients

- **1** cup coconut milk
- **¼** cup chia seeds
- **¼** cup cocoa powder
- **1** tablespoon maple syrup
- **½** teaspoon vanilla extract

Directions

Vigorously whisk the milk, chia seeds, cocoa powder, maple syrup, and vanilla extract in a medium bowl or storage container, being careful to incorporate any cocoa powder sticking to the sides and bottom.

Cover the chia pudding and refrigerate until thick and creamy, at least 4 hours, or preferably overnight.

Give it a good stir and divide into two servings. Enjoy with fresh coconut whip cream and berries, if desired.

---

[35] See Chia Pudding
https://upload.wikimedia.org/wikipedia/commons/8/83/Chia_Pudding.PNG

Chapter 11: How to Eat at Any Restaurant with Sugar Control in Mind

Ok, "great stuff, Chris," I hear you say. But how do you actually do this sort of thing on the fly in a restaurant? This chapter is all about answering that question with real-life examples from actual menus at restaurants I've eaten at in the last month while working on finishing this book. I'm going to walk through the actual menu and point out the "good" items on it and the "bad" items on it from a sugar control perspective.

I'm not going to name the specific restaurants here for many reasons, not least because you might be reading this book years after its 2025 publication. Most of these places are in New Orleans, Louisiana – the sugar capital of the United States. One of New Orleans's many nicknames is Sugar Town. Domino Sugar is based here. King Cake and beignets are woven into the culture – this is a place where just about everything has sugar in it.

It is also where I live, where my sugar first got out of control, and where I beat diabetes. I was born and spent my childhood in New York, so the phrase "If I can make it there, I can make it anywhere" is part of my lexicon. But when you think about sugar control, New Orleans is the place that phrase applies to.

Taqueria Sunrise

One of my wife's and my favorite places to eat is a Central American taqueria near our house. People who don't know better might call it a "Mexican Food" place, but the owners are from San Salvador. It's been there forever and is something of a fixture that everyone has eaten at. When our daughter was a baby, it was ideal – the food comes out fast and the wait staff is quick on the draw. As a parent, when you never know if any particular meal is going to end in a kid meltdown, it had a lot to offer. Not least of which is yummy "Mexican" food. The menu shown is their current menu as of 2025. As you can see it has the usual suspects on it: burritos, enchiladas, etc.

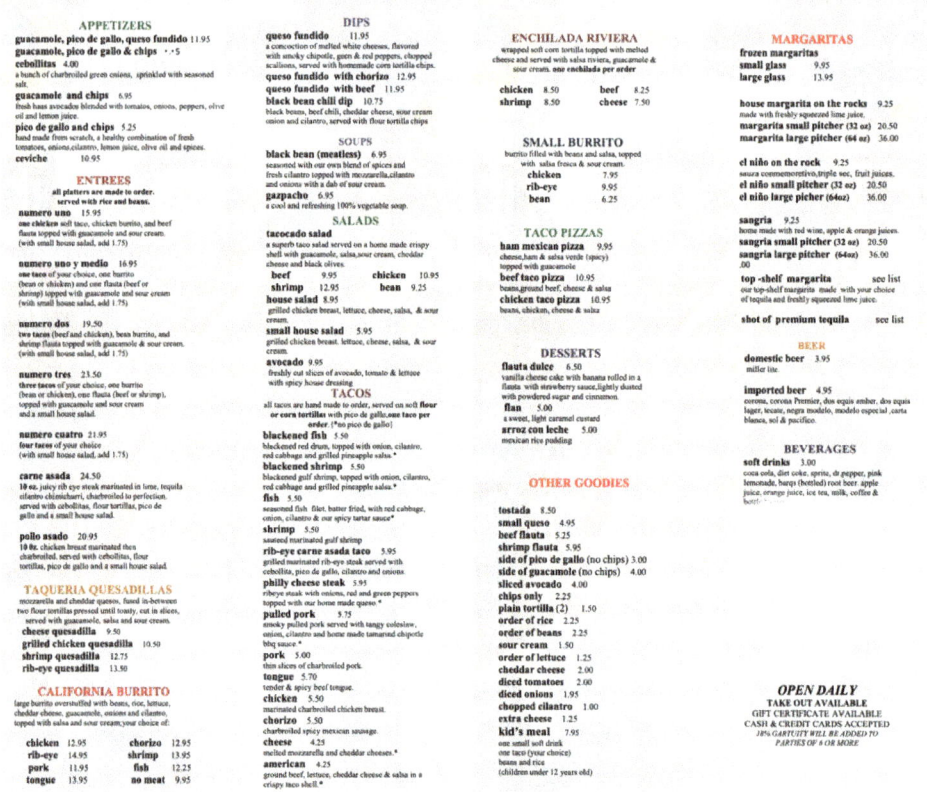

So, right away, let's concentrate on finding our friend, soluble fiber. Black beans feature heavily in Mexican and Central American cuisine – heck, beans of all sorts are pretty much a fixture. And beans, as we discussed previously, are a soluble fiber superstar. So instead of chips and pico de gallo (salsa), I order them with the bean dip. I make sure I get a lot of beans with each chip to maximize the value out of it.

But then there are some not-so-good items here too. Obviously, the rice is out, and those soft tacos made from flour are pretty much a no-go also. Sometimes I'll order a burrito and then eviscerate the thing – eating it with a fork and skipping that large flour wrap because it's just going to turn straight to sugar in my system.

But the "good" items don't end with the beans, although I do love refried black beans in general. Other good friends here are the fajitas – meat and peppers sizzling on a hot iron plate, and the tacos. If you get them "street" style, you just leave that flour tortilla underneath behind. With corn tortillas you're in a safer place – while there's usually some flour in them for stability, they're largely neutral from a sugar perspective.

As long as you skip the rice and flour tortillas, pretty much everything here is neutral or "good." I love fish tacos – grilled is obviously better than fried since that batter is mostly white flour.

Skip the dessert and obviously the soda, and you can eat here any day, easily avoiding sugar spikes while getting a delicious meal that's great for you.

Generally speaking, when I walk into a restaurant with folks I'm typically side-eying the sides and the appetizers. That is typically where I'll find the hit of soluble fiber that I'm looking for. And it is important to remember that as near as I can tell it is important to eat the soluble fiber foods first and the ones that may turn into sugar afterwards. I don't know enough about how digestion works on a micro-level like this but that certainly seems to make common sense to me. Certainly, I would be in favor of someone studying this effect to see if it is the case, but I eat like it is because that makes sense.

Rice Wine Café

My daughter's favorite sushi place is another uptown standby for us. This particular place has a lovely interior and a fantastic service staff. The sushi bar is quick, and they start with super high-quality, delicious ingredients.

But, as with all sushi places, rice is everywhere, and white rice is just no good for you if you're trying to control sugar spikes. I love white rice, and I love sushi, and since it's my daughter's go-to place, I eat there a fair bit.

As you can see from the menu, it's a pretty standard sushi place. All the usual items are here: rolls, sashimi, dumplings, and so forth. Nearly all of them are challenging from a sugar control standpoint.

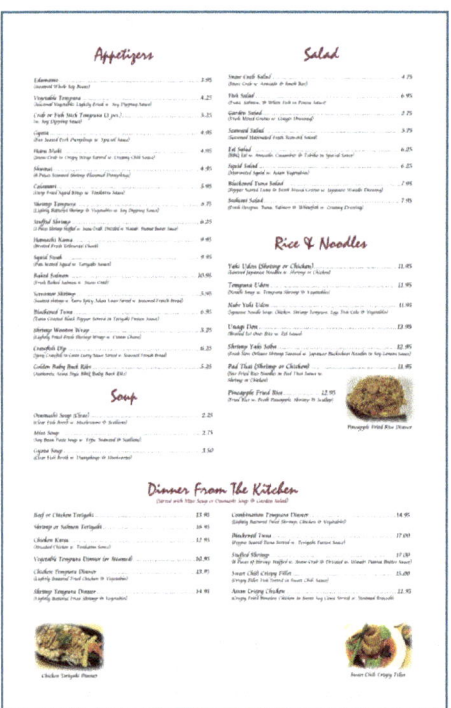
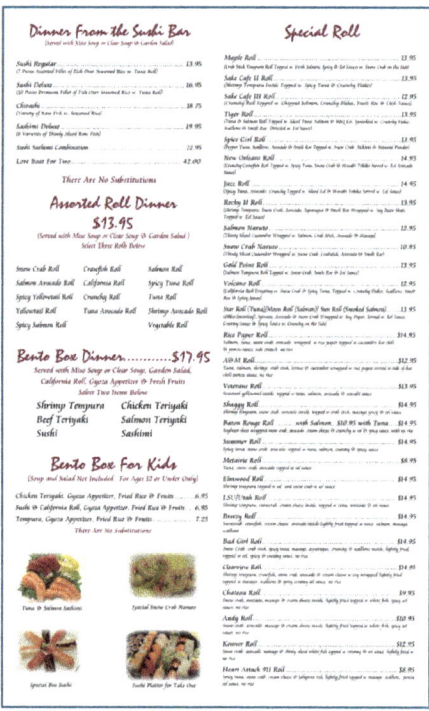

So, the things to avoid here are fairly obvious – white rice obviously but also gyoza, or flour dumplings with pork or other items inside. They're fantastic here but I can't order those. Instead I start with an entire order of edamame -

just for myself. I put down the whole thing and then order a roll. Dragon or crunchy are my two favorites. I also order nigiri (that's the fish on rice), usually tuna or salmon.

I eat the roll but with the nigiri I just take the fish and leave the rice. I suppose I could order sashimi instead but for whatever reason I like the nigiri better. Maybe it's because the fish is cut thicker?

Either way, we're going to take a sugar hit from the rice in the roll, which is unavoidable, but that's what the edamame was for!

The key here, and I hope this comes across clearly, is that soluble fiber can do a lot for you but if you overwhelm it with a ton of sugar-causing white rice, that magic is just not going to be enough: <u>an order of edamame is not going to offset four sushi rolls.</u>

Chimichango's

So this is a classic national chain. I don't eat there much since New Orleans is filled with amazing locally owned restaurants, but when traveling or if I have folks in from out of town, it is definitely an option.

It also gives us an opportunity to look at a place you find everywhere across the country and see what soluble fiber "friends" are on the menu.

The appetizers and sides are always good places to look for soluble fiber, and this menu is no exception. In the apps section, I'd stick with the guacamole and chips, eating as few chips as I can get away with. Guac is strong in soluble fiber, so it helps. It doesn't compete with broccoli or Brussels sprouts, but it's a great option here. Alternately, I might order the mozzarella sticks. It seems odd, and the breading is definitely not awesome from a sugar perspective, but it's the next "safest" item on this appetizer menu from how I see things.

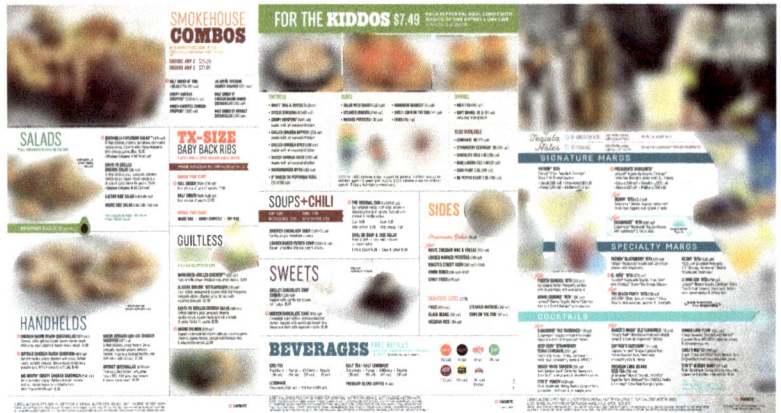

In the entrees, the steaks are strong if you order them with broccoli – definitely skip the fries or a baked potato. As much as I love, love, love a good baked potato, if you're working to control sugar they're just not a good idea. The Ancho Salmon and the Classic Sirloin with Avocado are also great options.

They also have black beans and broccoli available as sides with any dish. So you could do the Chicken Crispers and substitute the fries with broccoli or beans. The fajitas are also a good option if you either skip the tortillas entirely (which would be my choice) or go with corn tortillas. Make sure you eat the green peppers too if you order those though.

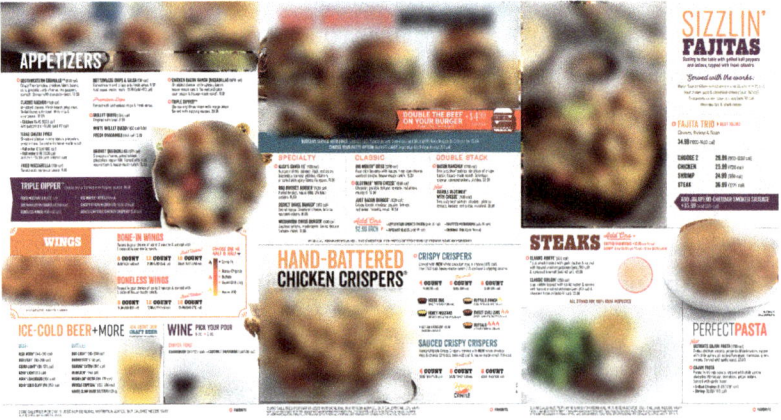

Georgiana's Tuscan Italian

This is a nice Italian restaurant near downtown. Very popular for dinner and a nice brunch spot as well.

When I take a look at this menu I see those good friends of mine, Brussels sprouts. I also see broccolini, which is like mini broccoli.

So, I'd order the Brussels as an appetizer or maybe the meatballs. I'd have the drum, pork or chicken.

I'd skip the pizza even though I love pizza, and if I wanted some pasta, I'd order either the campanelle" or the rigatoni and ask for it to be a little al dente. You may recall from the chapter on the glycemic index that al dente pasta actually has a pretty low GI.

I'd avoid the gnocchi even though I'm sure it's fantastic, because there is no way potato "pillows" are going to be good for me and you can't ask for your gnocchi "al dente."

If I didn't have the Brussels as an appetizer, I'd definitely order them or the broccolini as a side and make sure I ate those first. The entrees here are pretty good from a sugar standpoint, but I'd still try to front-load the fiber here.

MENUS
Lunch & Dinner Bar

ANTIPASTI

CHOPPED SALAD gem lettuce, salami, artichokes, olives, pickled peppers, red onion & parmesan	14
RIBOLLITA SOUP cannellini beans, parmesan, tomato, kale & fried ciabatta	12
FRIED CALAMARI basil & marinara	16
PROVOLA spicy sausage, provolone & oregano	13
MEATBALLS red gravy, parmesan & bread crumbs	12
CLAM TOAST marinated cherry tomatoes & sourdough	20
CIABATTA GARLIC BREAD chili butter & provolone	10

PRIMI

FENNEL SAUSAGE CAMPANELLE rapini, chili garlic & parmesan	18
RIGATONI AMATRICIANA guanciale, calabrian chili, tomato & pecorino	19
BRISKET AGNOLOTTI chestnut mushrooms, caramelized onion, tomato & pecorino	22
RICOTTA GNOCCHI beef bolognese & parmesan	20
ORECCHIETTE PESTO ALLA TRAPANESE shrimp, almond & pangrattato	22

PIZZA

MARGHERITA tomato, fior di latte & basil	22
SPICY SALAMI soppressata, mozzarella, tomatoes & banana peppers	24
MUSHROOM rosemary pesto, maitake mushrooms, provolone	24

ENTREES

DRUM ACQUA PAZZA tomatoes, capers, roasted fennel & herbs	32
LAMB LASAGNA braised lamb shoulder, mushrooms, bechamel & grana padana	36
GRILLED HALF CHICKEN olive tapenade & escarole	32
PORK MILANESE with lemon	36
16 OZ. PRIME RIBEYE marinated grilled onions	65

SIDES

FARM GREEN SALAD balsamic vinaigrette	10
BROCCOLINI garlic & anchovy breadcrumbs	12
PAESANO POTATOES rosemary, garlic & parmesan	8
WOOD OVEN BRUSSELS SPROUTS pepperoni & pecorino	10
PASTA BORDELAISE olive oil, garlic & parsley	8
WOOD OVEN FIRED PUCCIA BREAD rosemary & olive oil	8

DESSERT

BUTTERSCOTCH BUDINO with rosette cookie	12
LEMON MOUSSE CAKE with lemon anglaise & candied almonds	12
PANNA COTTA with seasonal fruit	12
GIANDUJA TART salted caramel & toasted hazelnuts	16
GELATO or SORBETTO with biscotti	7
LIMONCELLO lemon	7
ESPRESSO MARTINI vodka, montenegro, galliano ristretto	14

"Family Style" Eating and Ordering

Sometimes when you're eating out it is natural to order "family style," meaning that you order a whole bunch of entrees and appetizers and such and everyone shares in them and passes the serving dishes around.

This is fairly common in New Orleans, and I rather like it. It poses absolutely no problem in ordering for soluble fiber content, though. I just make sure that I order at least one of the dishes that is low in sugar content (usually a protein like chicken, fish, etc.). I then make sure we have some sides or apps that are soluble-fiber rich to make sure that I have those in there.

Typically speaking, nobody is jumping past me to grab the green beans, asparagus and broccoli so I'm usually getting the same stuff I would get if I ordered off the menu. And the plus of family style is that I get to try other options I might not have ordered otherwise.

Summary

I'm sure there's a restaurant not named McDonald's where I can't find soluble fiber, but thus far I have not found any. That said, one of the key things here is to forgive oneself for being human. I eat the way I eat to keep prescription drugs out of my life and to stay healthy as long as I can. I can't do that by making myself feel like crap if I can't find what I need on a menu.

In a pinch I'd eat as little as I could in a place with no fiber and make it up on the backside by doubling down the next day. I don't give myself a break, but I don't castigate myself either – I live in the real world where adverse-selection choices are everywhere. The key is the system and keeping to it – soluble fiber solves my sugar problems while also making me feel full and is good for me in other ways. I focus on that goal at all times – the rest just fades into the background.

Part V: Making These Changes Stick

Chapter 12: Habit Stacking and Virtue Bundling

This chapter is about sins and forgiveness and my two best friends in this journey: Habit-Stacking and Virtue-Bundling. Now, even though I grew up Catholic, I'm not big on guilt. But forgiveness? That I believe in – especially forgiving yourself for being human. I'll show you why this mindset is so crucial for pushing diabetes into remission and living a "normal" life.

Let's circle back to why I don't believe in dieting. Dieting is, by definition, a temporary measure. I'm arguing for a way to take control of your health and your life, and that can't be temporary if you want it to work. The methods I'm championing here aren't some temporary fix – they're a way of life that, once you get into it, becomes almost effortless.

Habit Stacking

Habit stacking is a way to make good habits stick by linking them to things you're already doing. Think of it as "stacking" something you should do onto something you definitely will do.

Here are a couple of examples how I use it to get myself to do stuff: I've got my Waterpik®[36] right in the shower, and while I'm waiting for my conditioner to do its thing (you know, those couple minutes it needs to work), I knock out the water pik as well as my stretching and shoulder PT exercises (volleyball player problems!). This isn't just about efficiency, though that's a nice bonus. It's about actually getting the good stuff done – the PT, the teeth cleaning, the stretching – by piggybacking them onto something I'm doing anyway, namely washing my hair.

The power isn't in multitasking; it's in making sure those healthy habits actually happen by tying them to your existing routines. There are hundreds of examples of good habit-stacking and many books and studies on the subject. I would be remiss if I did not footnote the person who introduced me to this idea, Angela Duckworth, from her celebrated podcast "No Stupid Questions."[37]

For sugar control, this means stacking up the lifestyle elements that are going to help you control your sugar levels with things that you already do. So, checking your glucose level while putting your clothes on as an example, so

---

[36] https://store.waterpik.com/
[37] See Episode 186 "Do You Need a Routine?"
https://freakonomics.com/podcast/do-you-need-a-routine/

that the small amount of wait time for the result coincides with the dead time of putting your socks and shoes on.

Temptation Bundling

Temptation bundling is a cousin to habit stacking. It's about pairing something that's good for you with a "treat" or indulgence. You saw this in action earlier when we talked about using soluble fiber to control sugar.

> You are not depriving yourself – you are making smart choices that let you have what you want.

Here's how it works: you "bundle" a big serving of hummus with your rice (half serving please), salad, and chicken shawarma. Those chickpeas in the hummus are packed with soluble fiber, helping offset the rice and pita bread. By bundling them together, you end up with a meal that's balanced from a sugar perspective. In my world, where I eat a lot of Middle Eastern food, I try to either ask for less rice or just skip it entirely.

Here's another example: you're at a steakhouse eyeing that yummy baked potato. Instead of skipping it entirely, you bundle it with a side of Brussels sprouts or broccoli, <u>making sure to eat those first</u>. This bundle is what makes the magic happen – it slows down digestion, keeps you feeling full longer, and prevents your sugar from spiking like it would if you just demolished the potato on its own.

But here's what's really beautiful about this approach: it lets you enjoy that baked potato without the guilt. You're not depriving yourself – you're making smart choices that let you have what you want. That's the real power of temptation bundling. For more info on temptation bundling and habit stacking see James Clear's book *Atomic Habits*,[38] which was an instant classic when it came out.

Clear takes a number of ideas that have been around for a long time and combines them into an easy-to-follow set of instructions. I find them invaluable. The Cleveland Clinic has a great summary article on these two ideas called "Everything You Need To Know About Habit Stacking for Self-Improvement."[39]

But how does this help? Why do it?

The reason I say I'm not suggesting or "selling" a diet, but rather a way to look at food and a way of living is because almost no one ever sticks to a diet – around 5% are still working on it a year later.[40] Nationally, a tiny percentage of people who start on a diet have regained weight that they lost when they were on their diet a year later.[41] Many have actually gained more weight, another bad marker for blood sugar and glucose health in my opinion.

Consider this – of all the diets the NIH studied in 2020, the Paleo Diet did the best – "The Paleo diet had the longest average compliance times among NJD (5.32 ± 0.68 weeks)". **That means that after just two months a majority had quit on the best diet out there!**

Similar issues abound for New Year's resolutions.[42] We just don't keep these "promises" to ourselves. Why? In my opinion diets and resolutions are

---

[38] See James Clear's website at https://jamesclear.com/
[39] See The Cleveland Clinic's "Everything You Need To Know About Habit Stacking for Self-Improvement " https://health.clevelandclinic.org/habit-stacking
[40] See USU article and summary of studies "The Dieting Dilemma" https://extension.usu.edu/nutrition/research/the-dieting-dilemma
[41] See the NIH study on this "How long do people stick to a diet resolution? A digital epidemiological estimation of weight loss diet persistence" https://pmc.ncbi.nlm.nih.gov/articles/PMC10200480/
[42] See The Pew Research Center "New Year's resolutions: Who makes them and why" https://www.pewresearch.org/short-reads/2024/01/29/new-years-resolutions-who-makes-them-and-why/

"sold" to us as a "fix" for what ails us. We think of them like a pill that you take and "everything" will be better. They are short-term and don't stick

This is why I don't believe in diets or deprivation or resolutions or promises. I believe in changing your view of food and its place in your world – once that new mindset takes hold you can never look at food the same way.

Here's the other thing that bugs me about diets: they're all about special foods, special timing, fasting rituals, and other short-term gimmicks. Sure, I made some radical changes to my eating when I started this journey to control my sugar and kick diabetes out of my life. But now? Even though I could probably ease up a bit, I find I don't even want to – this way of living has become so natural that most of the time I don't even think about it.

> I'm not going to lecture you about willpower or tell you to 'be strong' and just live with your cravings. Instead, I'm showing you how to actually have the things you want.

I've built these habit-stacks and virtue-bundles into my life so completely that they're just background noise now. It doesn't take effort because there's nothing special about it – soluble fiber-rich foods are everywhere (as you've seen throughout this book).

I never want to be that person asking for a special meal at restaurants. I don't need to hunt down exotic ingredients or shop at specialty stores.

What I did have to do was learn to spot soluble fiber opportunities everywhere – whether I'm scanning a menu, cruising the supermarket aisles, or even grabbing something at a 7-Eleven. Sure, that learning curve took some work, but once I got it? The rest was – and still is – easy.

Getting Started

Those first couple months of boosting my soluble fiber and controlling sugar were tough. I developed this crazy ability to smell sugar in everything (still can), and let's be real – I still love chocolate cake. I still get tempted by that warm bread the waiter brings to the table.

But here's what makes this approach different: I'm not going to lecture you about willpower or tell you to "be strong" and just live with your cravings. Instead, I'm showing you how to actually have the things you want. I won't demolish that massive slice of chocolate cake like I used to, and I'll skip the warm rolls (okay, maybe just one!), but if I have any of either, I'll balance it by loading up on soluble fiber from the appetizer menu. When they accidentally give me the sugared iced coffee now instead of the sugar-free one (I'm looking at you, Dunkin Donuts), I can't even drink it. It tastes heavy and "thick" and I don't want it.

The methods in this book aren't about denial – they're about smart choices that let you enjoy food while keeping your sugar under control. The fact that it also led to losing 10% of my body weight was a great benefit, but it's not what I was trying to do.

This way of living I'm sharing with you – the one I live every day – has completely changed how I perceive food. And you know what? It turned out to be for the better! I notice spices more now, and I try things I never would have before because I'm automatically scanning for those soluble fiber foods and making sure they're part of my meal.

Sometimes I slip up – sometimes my daughter waves an Oreo in front of me, and I end up eating four of them. But since I'm not "on a diet," I can forgive myself. I just make sure to boost my soluble fiber intake and move forward without beating myself up. I lean on my habit stacking and temptation bundling to navigate all my food choices throughout the day.

I truly believe anyone can do this in the same way that I don't think anyone can stick to a traditional diet. And that's exactly why this approach is worth following and why I had to write about it.

Chapter 13: Stress Management and Sleep

Mike Tyson famously said, "Everybody has a plan until they get punched in the face." Every diet survives until you have a deadline on a project or you're at a Mardi Gras parade and the King Cakes are laid out on the table in front of you. How we handle stress matters. How much and the quality of sleep that we get matters. These things play into how easy or hard it will be to keep our blood sugar under control.

This is because at the end of the day, your body responds to stress by putting other processes on hold and one of those things is cleaning up excess glucose.[43] It is believed that this form of hyperglycemia is caused by the "fight or flight" hormones from your sympathetic nervous system called cortisol and catecholamines.

Symptoms of Stress

We all know what it means to be "stressed out." Mostly it's around a particular incident ("I have to take the bar exam," "I'm getting married," "I just got a new job," and so forth). But it can also be a chronic thing that impacts your everyday life, and that's where we see the kinds of symptoms listed below.

Signs of stress:

- Trouble sleeping – this one really gets me
- Feeling unwell more and getting sick more than usual
- Digestive issues
- Depressive feelings – self medicating like drugs or alcohol
- Feeling angry and irritable

In a 2016 study,[44] it was found that "behavioral, psychological, and family processes that facilitate management of (stress) have been linked with improvements in A1c, suggesting the potential of interventions that strengthen positive processes to reduce stress and promote optimal glycemic control."

---

[43] Please see "What to know about stress hyperglycemia"
https://www.medicalnewstoday.com/articles/stress-hyperglycemia
[44] See Stress and A1c Among People with Diabetes Across the Lifespan
https://pmc.ncbi.nlm.nih.gov/articles/PMC4936828/

What the study essentially says is that being stressed out raises your glucose level and your resulting A1C readings. It quotes a 1998 study[45] that explains, "Over 60 years ago, Selye[1] recognized the paradox that the physiologic systems activated by stress can not only protect and restore but also damage the body." It is a great paradox – fight or flight adrenaline rushes are sometimes what keeps us alive, but if they go on too long, they damage and even kill us.

De-Stressors for Your Health

What does this mean for beating diabetes? High stress is not great. To be honest, it doesn't matter if you're diabetic or not – stress is just plain bad for you.

So what's a boy to do? What I do is try very hard to fit in 15-20 minutes of transcendental meditation (TM) daily. TM has been a godsend for me because it can be done anywhere at practically any time,

> I happen to be terrible about intrinsic motivation – I am happy to let me down all day.

doesn't take long, and drops my stress levels significantly. But I'm not here to shill for transcendental meditation – study after study shows that it doesn't really matter what type of meditation, mindfulness, prayer, yoga or whatever internally focused mental clearing you do. It matters that you can stick to it.[46]

---

[45] See Protective and damaging effects of stress mediators
https://scholar.google.com/scholar_lookup?journal=N%20Engl%20J%20Med&title=Protective%20and%20damaging%20effects%20of%20stress%20mediators&author=BS%20McEwen&volume=338&publication_year=1998&pages=171-9&pmid=9428819&doi=10.1056/NEJM199801153380307&

[46] See Meditation: A simple, fast way to reduce stress
https://www.mayoclinic.org/tests-procedures/meditation/in-depth/meditation/art-20045858

Because, at the end of the day, a meditation you like but you don't do regularly is almost worthless but a yoga class that you go to weekly, even though you don't like yoga, is priceless.

There are two types of motivation that are generally thought to exist. "Intrinsic," or motivation that comes from within, and "Extrinsic" which comes from external sources.[47] I happen to be terrible about intrinsic motivation – I am happy to let myself down all day. Sign me up for the gym and I'm happy to pay and not go (they're kind of counting on people like me).

But give me an extrinsic factor, like a friend who goes to yoga with me, a volleyball team I belong to or a coach that I schedule time for, and I'm 100% in. I'm old enough to know this about myself and so I lay "traps" for myself that force the behaviors that I am trying to get myself to do. This is kind of like temptation bundling, which we talked about in the previous chapter, but it's also its own thing. I use both – I'll use anything that gets me to do the things I really want to do done.

> **In summary: Meditation of any sort lowers your stress, which lowers your stress-related blood sugar spikes, which keeps down your A1C, and that's what we're trying to get done here.**

Mr. Sandman

Sleep is a problem in my life. I used to struggle to get to sleep – I'd toss and turn for hours sometimes. I tried everything: books, chamomile tea, you name it. The one thing that worked for me was watching the same movies over and over again. I had a VCR and TV in my bedroom and I watched *The Breakfast Club, Die Hard, The Princess Bride, Caddyshack* and some others literally hundreds and hundreds of times. Once I got something in rotation, I wouldn't make it ten minutes into the movie before I was out cold. It was

---

[47] See xtrinsic & Intrinsic Motivation Examples – What's the Difference? https://sprigghr.com/blog/hr-professionals/extrinsic-intrinsic-motivation-examples-whats-the-difference/

magical. And once I got to sleep, I was good at staying asleep. I would wake up and all would be better in the world.

When I was dating my now wife, and we moved into an apartment together, this became an issue. She falls asleep in about five minutes, if that. She stays asleep all night and is generally really well rested, curses upon her! She couldn't put up with my movies-to-go-to-sleep routine and banished the TV from the bedroom.

At first this was a disaster for my sleep. But then I discovered that I could do the same thing that I had done with movies, but now with books. So I've now read <u>all</u> of Agatha Christie's collected works, all of Sherlock Holmes, all of Tolkien, among other authors, over and over and over and over. I wish I didn't have to lull my brain into submission, but it is what it is.

I bring this up because getting a decent night's worth of sleep has a lot of benefits, and one of those many benefits is that you have better glucose control when you have better sleep. I quote the article covering a recent study about this:[48] "Scientists at the University of California, Berkeley, recently found that for some people, these waves could also serve as early warning signs of diabetes. The results, published in July in Cell Reports Medicine, suggest that getting a restful sleep may help control high blood sugar."

This seems to be because the hippocampus regulates a lot of our hormones and signaling across the entire brain and thus to our organs like the liver and pancreas. However, exactly what is going on here is not understood yet.

---

[48] See A Good Night's Sleep May Help Control Blood Sugar
https://www.scientificamerican.com/article/a-good-nights-sleep-may-help-control-blood-sugar/

Chapter 14: Exercise – the Great Cure-All

Exercise is Medicine

Which brings us to the other thing shown to reduce blood sugar and A1C – exercise. And it doesn't have to be serious, knock-it-all-out exercise. A great example of this is the 2017 study[49] demonstrating that small amounts of exercise after a meal really help.

> "Intermittent standing breaks throughout the day and after meals reduced glucose on average by 9.51% compared to prolonged sitting. However, intermittent light-intensity walking throughout the day saw a greater reduction of glucose by an average of 17.01% compared to prolonged sitting"

Because I believe in habit-stacking, I have started taking the dog for a walk around the block after dinner. We don't go far, and it takes about 5 minutes, but it really helps.

I'm a volleyball player – I've been playing for over 20 years and it is a big part of my life. Typically, I play three days a week. Sometimes it is super-intense exercise. But it appears that walking the dog after a meal is probably even better for me than playing 5 games of doubles on the sand courts. And that's not because walking the dog is better exercise or more fun – it's neither.

But it's something more important – timely. And by walking the dog right after dinner instead of sitting on the couch for those five minutes or answering my email, it makes a noticeable impact on my glucose level after a meal.

---

[49] See Just 2 minutes of walking after eating can help blood sugar, study says https://www.ncbi.nlm.nih.gov/search/research-news/17034/ and the actual study "The Acute Effects of Interrupting Prolonged Sitting Time in Adults with Standing and Light-Intensity Walking on Biomarkers of Cardiometabolic Health in Adults: A Systematic Review and Meta-analysis" at https://link.springer.com/article/10.1007/s40279-022-01649-4

The other consistent exercise after a meal that I have habit-stacked into my life is the morning coffee walk. My wife and I started doing this during the pandemic and it has really stuck hard.

What we do is have breakfast, but no coffee, and then walk to a coffee place that we really like, which is a little less than a mile away. It takes about 15 minutes. Sometimes we take the dog. We get coffee and drink it while we walk back home.

This gets my butt out of the house and walking early in the day right after I've had breakfast. If I make it to 90 it will probably be because of these walks, not because I got my heart rate up to 150 playing volleyball with people half my age, although that probably helps too. It also provides an opportunity for my wife and I to talk about random things going on and to just enjoy a walk together, which has its own benefits as well.

> The point here is that small amounts of effort, especially ones that are extrinsically motivated, can make a huge difference in how well you control sugar long-term and how healthy you are overall.

The point here is that small amounts of effort, especially ones that are extrinsically motivated or habit-stacked, can make a huge difference in how well you control sugar long-term and how healthy you are overall.

So much in the media and on TikTok and in magazines is telling people all these extreme exercise routines, diets and supplements that will make you healthy. But the truth, as revealed by quite a bit of science, is that small amounts of effort, if applied consistently, are worth more and are effective at a much higher rate than large efforts that people only make for a short period of time.

Mo' Exercise is Mo' Better

There are a lot of studies and meta-analyses (a study that surveys many other studies and combines the data) about exercise and sugar control. For example, I quote below one of these meta-studies,[50] called "Physical Activity/Exercise and Diabetes: A Position Statement of the American Diabetes Association." This is a survey of a bunch of studies about exercise and diabetes. The conclusion they come to is that overall, more exercise is better for sugar control.

Their quote, which I double-underlined myself, is that "aerobic exercise clearly improves glycemic control in type 2 diabetes, particularly when at least 150 min/week are undertaken Resistance exercise (free weights or weight machines) increases strength in adults with type 2 diabetes by about 50% and improves A1C by 0.57%."

> …aerobic exercise clearly improves glycemic control in type 2 diabetes, particularly when at least 150 min/week are undertaken. Resistance exercise (free weights or weight machines) increases strength in adults with type 2 diabetes by about 50% and improves A1C by 0.57%

What this means is that you can drop your A1C by about half a point by working out in some kind of aerobic activity about 2 hours per week and doing some weight lifting.

I happen to play volleyball but I could just as easily pick up pickleball or bike riding or any one of a hundred other things.

---

[50] Physical Activity/Exercise and Diabetes: A Position Statement of the American Diabetes Association
https://pmc.ncbi.nlm.nih.gov/articles/PMC6908414/#:~:text=Moreover%2C%20aerobic%20exercise%20clearly%20improves,by%200.57%25%20(64)

What this analysis is saying is that any exercise helps sugar control if you do enough of it. My suggestion, as always, is to get involved in something where other people are depending on you to show up. Nothing beats peer pressure to get your butt up and off to spinning class or to the tennis court.

Part VI: Additional Considerations

Chapter 15: Alcohol and Diabetes

Sing it with me people, Alcohol does **NOT** metabolize into sugar. This is the most common misconception people have about sugar and booze, probably because alcohol comes from sugars. But here's the real kicker for diabetics: the actual risk with alcohol isn't raising your blood sugar – it's lowering it.

This is a little complicated,[51] but the reality is that alcohol tends to create what's called a "yo-yo effect," which is actually more dangerous on the low-sugar end than the high. For Type 1 diabetics, this can be really dangerous. But from what I can tell, it's a pretty minor risk for most Type 2 diabetics – most of us can drink pretty much like we always have.

The bigger issue, from my perspective, is not the booze - it's what comes along with it. Mixers are the biggest issue if you like cocktails or mixed drinks. An old fashioned literally has simple syrup (aka glucose) as a primary ingredient. But pretty much 95% of the standard mixers you find in a bar are trouble. Orange juice in your champagne, simple syrup (the worst – it is literally liquid sugar) in your French 75 or a mojito. All of them are bad news. I love a margarita still, but they're pretty much off my drink menu nowadays because of the amount of fruit juice and sugar.

For me, I used to drink bourbon and ginger ale and in the '90s I liked gin and tonic. What I didn't realize was ginger ale is basically the same as Coca-Cola. Lots of calories and tons of sugar. Tonic is pretty much also the same – 42.9 grams of sugar in one of those little bottles of tonic water. That's about ten sugar packets, just in one little bottle.

So I switched to club soda as a mixer. And that's made quite a difference. Now, if I'm out with friends and someone accidentally gives me ginger ale as a mixer, it tastes so sickly sweet to me that I can't even imagine drinking it.

I tend to stay away from beer, especially those heavy ones like craft brews, stouts, and other carb-loaded beers. The official GI for beer is 70, which is high, but if you tested a low-carb light beer against a Guinness, you'd obviously see some huge differences.

Wine and Champagne

Wine is generally pretty good (glycemic index of zero to 15) and red wine can help with cholesterol. But Champagne is rated at 60 (probably what's added

---

[51] Please see "Diabetes mellitus and alcohol"
https://pubmed.ncbi.nlm.nih.gov/15250029/

to it) so I'd stick with chardonnay and stay away from the bubbly. To be frank, my experience with wine and sugar is fairly low, as I only drink wine occasionally and champagne even less.

So here's the bottom line: alcohol is really bad for type 1 diabetics because it can create that yo-yo effect and drop their sugar dangerously low – even to the point of diabetic coma. For type 2 or insulin resistant folks, yeah, you should take it easy on the booze for all kinds of reasons, but what's really critical is ditching those sugary mixers and staying away from champagne and heavy beer. Look, I know I'm living in a bit of a glass house here, but I'm absolutely religious about my mixers and I try to keep the day-drinking or nights out to a minimum.

Chapter 16: Supplements and Alternative Treatments

Berberine vs Metformin – experimenting on myself

For centuries, people have been using extracts from turmeric, barberry, goldenseal, and other plants as medicine. Because of this long history, the resulting formulations – often lumped together as berberine – are classified as dietary supplements rather than prescription medicines. A ton of research shows that berberine is just as effective as metformin. Metformin itself is really just distilled French lilac.[52] As with many medications, the line between medicine and herbal concoction or dietary supplement is a pretty fluid one.

I really wanted to be able to check that "no medications" box on every form in my life, so I did a personal experiment: six months of berberine versus six months of metformin. I tolerate both really well, like most people do. Sure, metformin is more likely to give some folks gas and stomach issues, and some people say the same about berberine. I got lucky – other than a brief adjustment period where I felt a little gassy, neither one bothered me at all.

In the end, they were identical in effect. My A1C didn't change in any significant way between berberine and metformin. But since berberine is officially classified as a supplement, not a drug, it makes a difference – I can truthfully say I'm not taking any drugs to control diabetes.

Personally, I hate that I even have to care about this. It's ridiculous that we stigmatize people this way, but that's life in the United States right now. Taking "supplements" is "ok" and not tracked as an indicator of bad health (and sometime even considered an indicated of good health), but taking "medications" is, even when often they're the same thing. So, in my world, if

---

[52] Please see "A second look at the ancient drug: new insights into metformin" https://pmc.ncbi.nlm.nih.gov/articles/PMC4200662/

you want the extra "help" that metformin gives you without technically taking "drugs," berberine might be your answer.

The only real downside I've found with berberine is having to take it twice a day - once in the morning and once at night. It's annoying, but pretty small beans in the grand scheme of things, so I deal with it.

Here's something interesting: even though metformin is a prescription drug, it's been around and off-patent for so long that it's actually cheaper than berberine for the same time period. The difference is small (we're talking a few bucks a month from the place I buy it), but it can add up over time. Either way you look at it, both are way cheaper than insulin or any of those thousands of other drugs out there.

The Elephant in the Room – Ozempic

I never tried Ozempic or any of those other "fancy" drugs because I never got that far. I started with Metformin, eventually got off even that, and now just throw down some Berberine. Look, I'm sure Ozempic helps lots of people, and I'm not here to knock it. It's pretty wild, though – it went from something nobody had heard of to being splashed across every news and diet website out there in less than a year.

However, cutting through all the b.s. (and there's a lot of it), from what I can tell, our old friend from the Direct Study (see Chapter 8) is showing up again – if you lose more than 10% of your body weight, odds are pretty good your diabetes will go into remission.[53] There are a lot of ways to get there. Let's face it, we Americans love our pills and quick fixes, so I'm sure Ozempic will continue to be a godsend for folks with Type 2 diabetes, and probably a whole lot more people who just want to drop a few pounds.

---

[53] Please see "Reversing Type 2 Diabetes and ongoing remission" https://www.ncl.ac.uk/magres/research/diabetes/reversal/#publicinformation

But here's where I'll put in a plug for my methods. Ozempic costs money – and not just a little. You also have to keep taking it forever to keep the weight off. You need a prescription. Bottom line? It's not that different from insulin – you're still tied to something you can't live without.

My method of eating soluble fiber and avoiding added sugar doesn't require you to buy any pills, and study after study and my own experience says if you stick to it, you will absolutely lose weight and keep it off as long as you keep eating fiber-rich foods.

No prescription needed, no permission required – you can do this completely on your own, without anyone even knowing. Those "Wow – you look great" comments and "When did you lose so much weight?" questions are great byproducts of living the way I've outlined in this book, but they're just side effects. Beating diabetes without taking medicine is the goal, but this approach has so much more to offer for your overall health.

Chapter 17: Healthcare Providers – the Scarlet Letter "D"

When I got that first reading of a high A1C I immediately read up on everything. I had what seemed to be Rapid-Onset Diabetes, which has a slightly less than 1% chance of being pancreatic cancer,[54] which at 46 would likely have killed me within 14 months on average.

---

[54] See https://www.cancer.gov/news-events/cancer-currents-blog/2021/pancreatic-cancer-diabetes-early-detection. Relevant quote here: "Out of 10,000 participants, Drs. Chari and Maitra estimate that about 85 will develop pancreatic cancer..."

To say I was freaked out is a massive understatement – the more I read, the scarier the reading got. I insisted on having an MRI to see if I had pancreatic cancer. The internist I went to said "Do you know how unlikely that is?" when I asked him to do the test.

"Yes, just under 1%. I don't want to be Mr. 1% here."

An important detail here – my mother was an actuary who specifically worked on large-scale healthcare plans, so I grew up very aware of how the insurance industry views people with Type 2 diabetes. I also knew that this "progressive, incurable" disease represents huge costs to the insurance industry.

Lastly, and maybe most importantly, I learned that an official diagnosis of Type 2 diabetes is when you have a second test within a few months with A1C over 7[55] confirmed by a doctor. I was hell-bent that there would never be a second test where my A1C was over even 6.

So, I made the hardest left-turn of my life – cut every single kind of sugar out, tested my blood obsessively, and ordered home A1C tests to track my progress. Looking back, I was probably a little over the top and didn't need to go quite that crazy.

But it worked. I fired my primary care physician and got a nutritionist and a concierge doctor instead. Yeah, it was a little costly, but I figured my whole life depended on this – which, in many ways, it probably did. With my concierge doctor's help, some guidance from the nutritionist, and a ton of research (most of which I've shared in this book), I got my A1C down to 6 within 30 to 40 days and to 5.5 within 3 months. And here's the kicker: I haven't had an A1C test over 5.7 in the 7+ years since.

---

[55] See Classification and Diagnosis of Diabetes: Standards of Medical Care in Diabetes—2022
https://diabetesjournals.org/care/article/45/Supplement_1/S17/138925/2-Classification-and-Diagnosis-of-Diabetes

I'm not telling this story to pat myself on the back, although I am proud of the effort and discipline I put in. I'm telling it because in our country, a diabetes diagnosis is treated like MS or Parkinson's, but without a "Race for the Cure." There's zero expectation of any way out – the medical and insurance establishments take it as gospel that nobody, not you, not me, not anyone, can reverse or eliminate diabetes once it's been "diagnosed."

This scarlet letter D scared me enough to put herculean efforts into keeping it from ever being sewn into my medical chart.

But most people don't know these are the consequences of such a diagnosis. Most don't even realize that the second A1C test is the critical one. Few believe there's another answer.

For over seven years, I've kept my first test a secret. Only my doctors, close friends, and a couple of co-workers know this story. It scares me, honestly, to write it down and publish this book – because I know there will be those who'll say I'm fooling myself, that in the end diabetes will come back and get me.

The future is a crystal ball – who can say they aren't right? But I know I live the way I live now and keep my sugar 100% under control with what seems like almost no effort anymore.

Yeah – I ordered the veggie platter with green beans and broccoli at the Indian restaurant last night. But I also had the Butter Chicken that I went there for. Balancing that bit of white rice with the veggies hardly seems like a burden anymore, and I know that because of the way I live – the way I've written about in this book – I'm far healthier, happier, and will very likely live a lot longer than if I'd kept living the way I used to.

Jim Morrison put it perfectly, as he did so many times, "Nobody gets out of here alive." But what he missed is that how you live is critical – your relationship with the basic things in your life – that makes all the difference.

I hope, with all my heart, that what I've shared here will help others do what I did: beat diabetes, or at least push it into remission, with little or no drugs. If this effort helps my friend Tim, who inspired me to write it all down, that's great. If it goes beyond that and helps more people, that would exceed my wildest hopes.

Thank you for reading my manifesto about beating diabetes. If you find it useful, please spread the word.

Chris Reade
Winter 2024

As a footnote to this story, I recently had Tim and his family over for Thanksgiving dinner. He'd dropped 80 pounds and his A1C was 4.9. The credit goes to him and especially to his wife for changing the foods in their house and what she cooks (she's famous in our friend group for her creole-style cooking). "Food is medicine" as they say, and Tim shows that you can put this book to practical and effective use.

You can read more about Beating Diabetes at https://BeatingDiabetes.us

Beating Diabetes
By: Christopher Reade
© 2024 LookFar Ventures LLC and Christopher Reade, All Rights Reserved

ISBN: 979-8-9927456-0-3

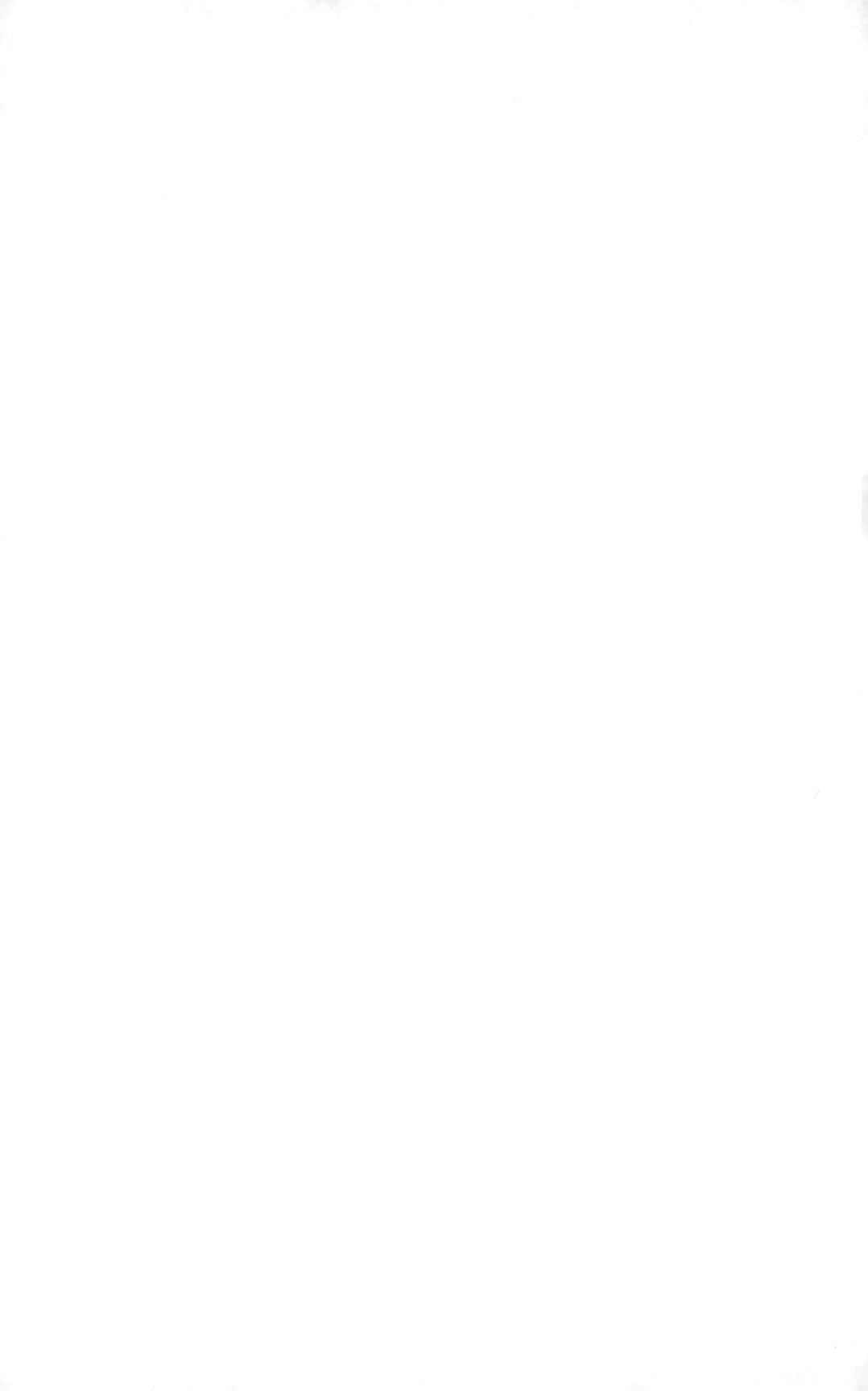

www.ingramcontent.com/pod-product-compliance
Lightning Source LLC
Chambersburg PA
CBHW060504030426
42337CB00015B/1732